Ethics, Law and the Veterinary Nurse

For Elsevier:

Commissioning Editor: Mary Seager
Development Editor: Rebecca Nelemans
Project Manager: David Fleming
Designer: Andy Chapman
Illustration Manager: Bruce Hogarth

Ethics, Law and the Veterinary Nurse

Edited by

Sophie *Pullen* BSc(Hons) CertEd VN

Carol *Gray* BVMS MRCVS

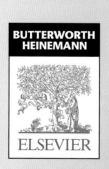

BUTTERWORTH
HEINEMANN

ELSEVIER

Edinburgh   London   New York   Oxford   Philadelphia   St Louis   Sydney   Toronto   2006

BUTTERWORTH
HEINEMANN
ELSEVIER

First published 2006

ISBN 10: 0 7506 8844 0
ISBN 13: 978 0 7506 8844 4

British Library Cataloguing in Publication Data
A catalogue record for this book is available from the British Library

Library of Congress Cataloging in Publication Data
A catalog record for this book is available from the Library of Congress

Knowledge and best practice in this field are constantly changing. As new research and experience broaden our knowledge, changes in practice, treatment and drug therapy may become necessary or appropriate. Readers are advised to check the most current information provided (i) on procedures featured or (ii) by the manufacturer of each product to be administered, to verify the recommended dose or formula, the method and duration of administration, and contraindications. It is the responsibility of the practitioner, relying on their own experience and knowledge of the patient, to make diagnoses, to determine dosages and the best treatment for each individual patient, and to take all appropriate safety precautions. To the fullest extent of the law, neither the publisher nor the author assumes any liability for any injury and/or damage.

The Publisher

Working together to grow
libraries in developing countries

www.elsevier.com | www.bookaid.org | www.sabre.org

ELSEVIER   BOOK AID
International   Sabre Foundation

your source for books,
journals and multimedia
in the health sciences
www.elsevierhealth.com

The
Publisher's
policy is to use
**paper manufactured
from sustainable forests**

Printed in China

Contents

Contributors

Sophie Pullen BSc(Hons) CertEd VN
Director, 2by2 Training, East Sussex, UK
Nurse Administrator, Rossdales Equine Hospital, New Market, Suffolk, UK

Siobhan Mullan BVMS MRCVS DWEL
Senior Clinical Scholar in Animal Welfare Science, Ethics and Law,
University of Bristol, Bristol, UK

Carol Gray BVMS MRCVS
Lecturer in Veterinary Communication Skills, University of Liverpool,
Liverpool, UK

Kathryn Wilson LL.B DipLP
Associate, Melrose and Porteous Solicitors, Duns, Berwickshire, UK

Elizabeth Earle BA RGN Cert Ed
Head of Veterinary Nursing, Royal College of Veterinary Surgeons,
London, UK

Sally Bowden BSc(Hons) CertEd VN
Director, 2by2 Training, East Sussex, UK
Senior Veterinary Nurse, Wylie Veterinary Centre, Essex, UK

Pippa Swan BVSc CertWEL MRCVS
Animal Welfare Consultant, RL Consulting, Oxford, UK

Giles Legood BD MTh DMin AKC
Chaplain and Honorary Lecturer in Veterinary Ethics, Royal Veterinary
College, London, UK

Kirstie Dye MPhil PGCHE BSc(Hons) RGN
Senior Lecturer, School of Health and Social Sciences, Middlesex
University, Enfield, UK

Gordon Hockey MRPharmS, Barrist er
Head of Professional Conduct
Assistant Registrar, Royal College of Veterinary Surgeons, London, UK

Tania Dennison BSc(Hons) BVMS MRCVS
Clinical Training Scholar in Equine Welfare, University of Bristol, Bristol,
UK

Matthew Leach BSc(Hons) MSc PhD
Researcher, Department of Clinical Veterinary Science, University of
Bristol, Bristol, UK

Dympna Crowley RN RM RNT MA
Senior Lecturer, Middlesex University, Royal Free Campus, Royal Free
Hospital, London, UK

Foreword
Dot Creighton

Veterinary nursing is continually evolving and strengthening its position as a veterinary profession, with a unique and fundamental role in the health and welfare of animals.

We have reached yet another turning point as the reality of a regulated veterinary nursing profession and all this entails approaches. The RCVS Veterinary Nurses Council is currently developing a non-statutory regulatory framework, while at the same time the RCVS are preparing for a new Veterinary Surgeons Act. There is uncertainty as to when this will come into force but inevitably will dictate the start of statutory regulation for veterinary nurses.

In the meantime, a code of conduct is being written specifically for veterinary nurses to give detailed guidance on what is expected of a professional who will be personally accountable, and within the terms of new legislation, legally accountable for their actions. An emphasis on animal welfare being of primary consideration, respecting the clients wishes, the need to develop our professional knowledge and skills as well as upholding the integrity of the veterinary nursing profession not only to our colleagues but also to the general public, will necessitate a detailed understanding of many unexplored subjects such as confidentiality and informed consent, as well as the implications of delegation, negligence and whistle blowing.

Such a book is therefore timely as it introduces veterinary nurses to law and ethics and how it applies to them and their working environment. The chapters that follow give a fascinating insight into these subjects as well as giving veterinary nurses the confidence to professionally discuss, question and challenge some of the situations they find themselves in. I quote from one of Carol Gray's chapters, '. . . a working knowledge of the law can enhance the veterinary nurses role in practice . . .'. This applies to knowledge of both law and ethics.

Ethics, law and the Veterinary Nurse will help veterinary nursing students develop an understanding of regulation as they train and prepare for their future and will be crucial to many qualified veterinary nurses as a much needed starting point, ahead of change. Sophie Pullen and Carol Gray, both highly respected in the veterinary and veterinary nursing profession, have edited this book to provide the reader with an informative and thought provoking text and fill a much needed gap in our knowledge and understanding.

Dot Creighton VNDipAVN (surgical)
Vice-Chair RCVS Veterinary Nursing Council
BVNA Past President and Honorary Member

Preface

Veterinary nurses encounter ethical and moral dilemmas in their everyday work. This book sets out to introduce the concept of ethical thinking and decision-making within the current legal framework. Some chapters include the authors' personal opinions, but these are included to encourage debate and reflection on current practice.

Procedures such as spaying pregnant cats and euthanasing healthy animals are situations that veterinary nurses sometimes have to face in their career. A student veterinary nurse once commented that she felt really upset when asked to assist in performing what she referred to as an 'abortion' on a cat. Having mentioned this to the practice principal she was informed that it was 'her job' and what she was 'paid to do'. Is there a place for personal ethics in veterinary practice?

Advances in knowledge and technology mean that veterinary surgeons are now performing procedures that would not have been thought possible a few years ago, such as total hip replacements. They are also better able to prolong the life of animals by using new drug combinations, for example, different chemotherapy protocols for the treatment of cancers. Their ability to undertake these procedures does not make them 'right' and in some instances, a veterinary nurse may have strong objections to a procedure.

By providing a comprehensive introduction to ethical theories, this book will allow constructive evaluation of moral issues, thereby empowering veterinary nurses and giving them the confidence to challenge accepted practices.

In an attempt to complement other veterinary nursing textbooks we have been selective in our choice of legal topics and have concentrated on those areas that we believe to have important influence on the future of the profession. We also acknowledge that there are imminent changes to some important legislation (for example, the Animal Welfare Bill, and a review of the Veterinary Surgeons Act).

Expectations of veterinary practice are changing. We no longer live in a society that accepts that mistakes happen and no one is to blame. Clients expect high standards from practice, and as a result, if things go wrong, they will seek explanations and resolutions. It is for this reason that veterinary nurses need to understand the protocols and reasons behind issues such as informed consent. It is no longer enough to 'get the client to sign the form'.

Animal welfare is central to the veterinary nursing profession, therefore knowledge of the law in this area is crucial. We have included legislation on the use of animals in research, as it is anticipated that veterinary nurses will become more involved in the research process as the profession develops.

It must be appreciated that becoming a complete veterinary nurse is not just about acquiring knowledge and perfecting clinical techniques. It is also about learning how to question attitudes and values, by developing critical and reflective skills. It is this aim that should be paramount to the profession as it approaches regulation. To this end, we have included some scenarios for you to consider. These appear in Appendix 1.

Finally, in writing this book, we hope to infect the reader with the same enthusiasm for the subjects of ethics and law as we have. You may not share our opinions, but if we can start you thinking about, and debating, the issues involved, we will have gone a long way towards achieving our goal.

Carol Gray and Sophie Pullen

Acknowledgements

This book would not have been possible without the help of the following people. We would like to thank them all very much.

Alison Watkins, Angela Maraconda and Lisa Brett, from the BVNA headquarters in Harlow, who answered queries, sent information and provided advice in such a friendly and efficient way.

Jane Hern, Registrar of The Royal College of Veterinary Surgeons, who assisted with the completion of Chapter 5 and provided the authors with information and advice.

The Library staff at the RCVS for helping to find references and dig out information as required.

Nicky Ackerly, HR Support Consultancy, for clarifying issues in relation to representation.

Lynne Henshaw, Lecturer at Middlesex University, for taking the time to discuss research ethics in relation to humans.

Jean and Trevor Turner, who provided an enormous amount of information in relation to the history of the profession. Thank goodness for people who save everything!

Melanie Roberts for her help with the information on Scots law.

Rebecca Nelemans and Mary Seager for their patience, help and support.

And finally to Sylvie Pullen for making sure that our sugar levels were maintained!

Acknowledgements

1
Veterinary nursing: the road to professionalism
Sophie Pullen

This is an exciting time for veterinary nurses! Moves to make veterinary nursing a regulated profession, together with proposed changes to the Veterinary Surgeons Act, are not only paving the way for an improved standard of animal welfare, but also increasing recognition for the profession.

With regulation comes accountability, and veterinary nurses must be conscious of what this will actually mean to them on a personal level and to the profession as a whole. Veterinary nurses need to be aware of the implications of autonomous practice and be prepared to meet the challenges that this will bring.

The purpose of this chapter is to examine the role of the veterinary nurse throughout the history of the profession, with a view to challenging opinions and perceptions and reviewing and evaluating the need for change. While readers may not agree with all that is discussed, it is hoped that they will appreciate the reasons why, now more than ever before, veterinary nurses need to develop an awareness of ethical principles and an understanding of the legal framework that governs the profession, and the treatment and management of the animals in their care.

THE INTRODUCTION OF VETERINARY NURSING

Although one can find references to companion animal nurses in the late 1800s it was not until the late 1940s and early 1950s, when small animal practice became an accepted part of British veteri-

nary practice, that the advantage of having qualified staff working within practice was realised.[1]

It was thanks to a few members of the British Small Animal Veterinary Association (BSAVA) that the training scheme for small animal nurses was launched in 1961. They identified the benefits of having veterinary nurses that were trained to a certain standard, and despite reservations by some members of the veterinary profession, they made successful representations to the Royal College of Veterinary Surgeons (RCVS).

Unfortunately, the term 'nurse' could only be used to describe persons working within human medicine, as the title was protected by nursing legislation at that time. As a result, the title of Registered Animal Nursing Auxiliary (RANA) was given to those persons who satisfied the requirements of the training scheme. The first Registered Animal Nursing Auxiliaries (RANAs) qualified in 1963. It was not until 1984, twenty-three years after the establishment of the first recognised qualification, that the title of RANA was changed to Veterinary Nurse (Fig. 1.1 and Table 1.1).

The evolving role of the veterinary nurse

As Pamela Pitcher, the first RANA to qualify, remembers, trainee nurses at that time had very little support. There were no animal nursing textbooks, no lectures and no guidelines to follow. There was no syllabus. Veterinary surgeons and laboratory staff assisted her, but much of the information she gained was through

Table 1.1 Major events in the history of veterinary nursing

Date	History
1961	The RCVS launched the first training scheme.
1963	The first Registered Animal Nursing Assistants qualified.
1965	The British Veterinary Nursing Association was inaugurated.
	Details of the 'uniform' approved by the BSAVA/RANA committee and by the RCVS were published. Veterinary Nursing green is still popular today.
1966	The title of the British Veterinary Nursing Association (BVNA) was changed to the British Animal Nursing Auxiliaries' Association (BANAA) as the title of 'nurse' was protected.
	The first edition of Jones's Animal Nursing was published.
1967	The Veterinary Record introduced a separate appointments section for veterinary nurses within the journal.
1968	A representative from BANAA was invited to serve on the RCVS/ANA Committee.
1970	BANAA issued its first newsletter. The forerunner to the Veterinary Nursing Journal (VNJ).
1974	The first BANAA congress was held at the Russell Hotel in London.
1981	The minimum entry requirement to the course was raised from 3 to 4 passes at O Level or grade 1 CSE.
1984	On the 1st November this year the title RANA was changed to Veterinary Nurse. This came about as the legislation governing the title 'nurse' was up for repeal.
	Rita Hinton became the first Veterinary Nurse to become president of the BANAA.
1985	BANAA reverted back to BVNA.
1988	The BVNA moved into its first official headquarters at the Seedbed Centre in Harlow.
1991	The Veterinary Surgeons Act 1966 was amended and the role of the veterinary nurse was formally recognised in law (Schedule Three).
	A 'list' of veterinary nurses was established by the RCVS as required by the Schedule Three amendment to the VS Act.
	The NVQ/SNVQ in Veterinary nursing was launched.
1992	The first cohort of veterinary nurses graduated with an Advanced Veterinary Nursing Diploma (Surgical).
2000	The first Equine Veterinary Nurses Qualified.
2002	The RCVS VN Council held its first meeting. The first cohort of students to complete the BSc honours programme in veterinary nursing graduated.
	The first cohort of veterinary nurses graduated with an Advanced Veterinary Nursing Diploma (Medical).
	Schedule Three of The Veterinary Surgeons Act 1966 was further amended so increasing the scope of the veterinary nurse's role (Appendix 1).

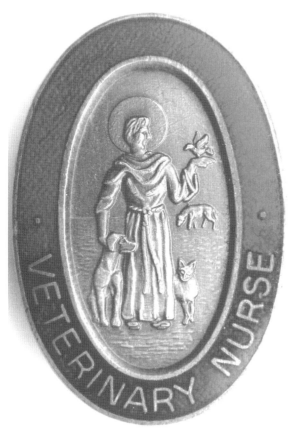

Figure 1.1 **Veterinary Nurse badge.** Pictured is St Francis of Assisi (born Giovanni Bernadone) 1182–1226. St Francis is the patron saint of ecologists and is well known for his ability to charm wild animals. His feast day is the 4th October.

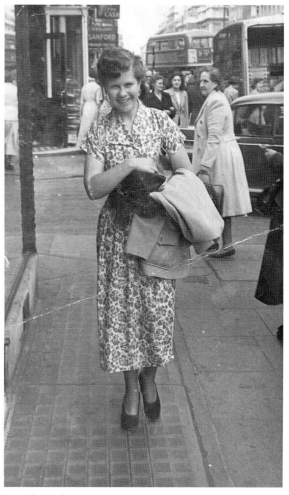

Pamela Pitcher

reading textbooks on veterinary surgery and human nursing.[2]

As a result, it is suggested that the nursing care given to patients was, at that time, based on the traditional 'medical model of nursing care'. A sentiment reinforced by Earnshaw in 1966, who stated that 'the legal liability of the RANA is that of a servant or employee . . . she has certain responsibilities towards her employer; to safeguard and further his interest . . . to behave carefully towards his clients remembering that her employer will have some liability for whatever actions she may perform during the course of her employment'.[3]

the patient, as far as possible, to full activity of normality',[4] the focus being 'cure' rather than 'care'.

The model describes a process where a veterinary surgeon and veterinary nurse work together to diagnose and treat a disease. The veterinary surgeon carries out an examination and performs various diagnostic tests and once a diagnosis has been made formulates a treatment plan. The veterinary nurse assists the veterinary surgeon throughout the process by, for example, collecting samples, performing laboratory tests, taking radiographs and administering prescribed treatments. The actions of the veterinary nurses are dictated by the requirements of the veterinary surgeon.

The nursing approach, using this model, is often 'task-orientated' whereby each nurse is given a particular responsibility. For example, one nurse may measure TPR (temperature, pulse and respiration) for all the patients, whilst another may be responsible for the fluid and food intake. This means that a number of different nurses may 'care' for the patient, thus making it difficult for one nurse to develop an holistic approach to the patient.

Veterinary nurses using this model may be referred to as 'hand maidens', a term that was commonly used within the field of human nursing to describe the nurse who helps the doctor and carries out orders whilst demonstrating no autonomy. The veterinary nurse is subservient to the veterinary surgeon as the patient 'belongs' to the veterinary surgeon.

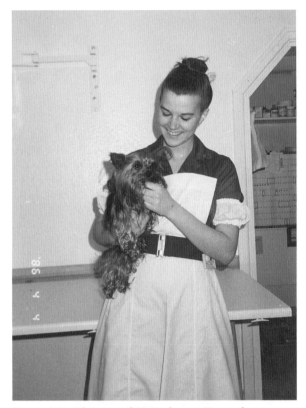

Figure 1.2 **Picture of Veterinary Nurse in uniform.** 'The nurse should be of clean and neat appearance at all times. Overalls, aprons and other protective clothing must be laundered frequently and always fresh; shoes should receive special attention and rubber boots must be washed frequently and always on removal. Hair should be controlled by means of a band or cap; hands must be always clean and fingernails should be kept short and well scrubbed. Outer garments should be neat, simple and free from "fuss" and jewellery of all kinds is out of place when on duty.'[4]

This model demonstrates the paternalistic, hierarchical structure which currently dominates the veterinary profession. An article on ethics for veterinary nurses, written as recently as 1989, contains the following: 'I was trained to respect the veterinary surgeon, the then RANA, the veterinary student and my own equals and treat those junior to me with consideration.'[5] This suggests that unquestioning respect is due to certain people by virtue of what they are rather than what they do.

In 1966 the first edition of Jones's Animal Nursing was published. This was the first book to be written specifically for those wishing to train as animal nursing auxiliaries and was designed around the syllabus. It was written by thirteen veterinary surgeons and one veterinary academic, highlighting the point that veterinary nursing continued to be driven by the veterinary profession, despite the fact that the first RANAs had now been qualified for three years. (Fig. 1.2)

It was not until the title of the book was changed to 'Veterinary Nursing' in 1994 that a veterinary nurse became involved in editing the book, an initiative that represented the greater role that the veterinary nurse had in the training and examination systems at that time. The book now boasted eight veterinary nurse authors, most having obtained further qualifications in the form of the Diploma in Advanced Veterinary Nursing or the Certificate in Education.

It is suggested that this book inspired and gave confidence to other veterinary nurses to write, and may have introduced publishers to the fact that veterinary nurses could become more involved in the production of books relating to their profession. Ten years on, the range of textbooks available to both student and qualified veterinary nurses has dramatically increased. One only has to look at the bookshelves in college libraries to witness the selection available. Veterinary nurses are increasingly becoming involved in writing and editing these books, a shift that demonstrates that veterinary nurses are beginning to take the initiative, and are becoming more involved in their profession.

The current situation

During the past twenty-four years many initiatives have been taken to improve the image and role of the veterinary nurse (see Table 1.1) and the profession has much to be proud of. However, one issue that veterinary nurses continue to face is the overriding influence still exerted on their profession by veterinary surgeons. Although this may be seen as 'kindly paternalism,' anecdotal evidence suggests that many veterinary nurses now see this continuing influence as a wish to dominate. Those veterinary nurses are keen to establish themselves as members of a profession in their own right and want to be able to direct and be responsible for their actions and their future. This point is highlighted by the results from the RCVS consultation paper in 2003, which indicated that 88% of nurses agree that regulation is necessary, if veterinary nursing is to develop as a profession.[6] So how would this work?

When discussing a similar situation within the field of human nursing, Faulkner[7] stated that,

despite the differences in role between the doctor and the nurse, it was important to ensure that there was close collaboration between the professionals so that there could be an ethos of professional sharing without a threat to either group. She went on to say that in order for this to occur, each had to 'earn the respect of the other' and each had to 'accept the unique role of the other.' The difficulty is that at the moment veterinary nurses do not have a definition of their role.

DEFINING THE ROLE OF THE VETERINARY NURSE

'There are many points of animal nursing which cannot be assessed by a written examination: a real love for all animals is essential of course; while some of the finest attributes any nurse can possess are concerned with speed and efficiency. When order has to be made out of the chaos that inevitably exists in a daily battle against time, the veterinary surgeon is solving one of his greatest problems if he searches for those qualities in a new recruit which will help him to beat the clock. If the would-be nurse possesses unshakeable calm, an inexhaustible supply of energy, and a good memory, she will certainly need them; not to mention the tact, incorruptible ethics and perfect grooming required by every good receptionist. Having found this angel, it would be reasonable not to expect her to scrub the surgery floor or to clean out a kennel, so another virtue must be added to the list – versatility.'[8]

This quotation, examining the qualities of a veterinary nurse, gives us an insight into what was expected of a veterinary nurse a year after the first training scheme was launched, over forty years ago.

During the past few years the role of the veterinary nurse has received much attention. Lectures have been presented, and articles written; however, the question: are veterinary nurses 'nurses' or are they 'mini-vets'? remains unanswered.

In order to examine this question further, we need to look at the role of a veterinary nurse in practice. Evidence suggests that veterinary nurses have a number of different roles within the practice setting. These are (Fig. 1.3):

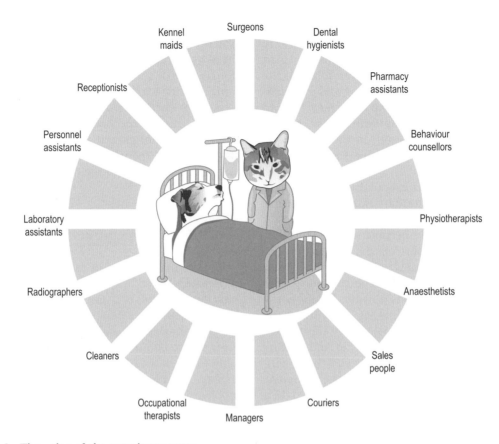

Figure 1.3 **The roles of the veterinary nurse.**

But are veterinary nurses nursing?

As the role of a veterinary nurse is still undefined we need to look to other professions in order to find out what the word 'nursing' actually means. The Royal College of Nursing, the representative body for nurses, defines nursing as 'the use of clinical judgement in the provision of care to enable people to improve, maintain, or recover health, to cope with health problems, and to achieve the best possible quality of life, whatever their disease or disability, until death'.[9]

This definition can easily be altered to suit the veterinary nurse by changing the focus from people to animals, however, is it one that could be adopted by veterinary nurses at this present time? In order to consider this further, we need to examine the definitions of 'clinical judgement' and 'care'.

Clinical judgement infers that nursing involves a process of decision-making. This is a concept that currently is not afforded to veterinary nurses as

they 'are only permitted to act under the supervision or direction of a veterinary surgeon'.[10] Veterinary nurses cannot therefore use their clinical judgement.

If nurses are unable to use clinical judgement do they provide nursing 'care'? Are veterinary nurses 'caring' for their patients?

Younger described caring as 'a function of the whole person in which concern for the growth and well-being of another is expressed in an integrated application of the mind, body and spirit toward maximizing positive outcomes in the one who is cared for' and goes on to add that 'human caring . . . is necessary for professional caring but it is far from sufficient'.[11] Thompson, Melia and Boyd concur with this sentiment and add that the difference between lay nursing and professional nursing is that professional caring requires not only caring and scientifically based knowledge, but also the use of methods validated by research,[12] a point reiterated by Younger who states that 'without professional competence it is not professional caring'.[11]

On the basis of this information it would appear that veterinary nurses are not caring for their patients in a nursing context, as they do not have the evidence base to allow them to do so. It is therefore suggested that, at the current time, the veterinary nurse is performing the role of a 'mini-vet'.

A veterinary surgeon could be defined as someone who diagnoses disease in animals; gives advice based upon such diagnosis; provides medical or surgical treatment for animals and performs surgical operations on animals.[13] A mini-vet could therefore be defined as someone who performs the same function as a veterinary surgeon, but to a lesser extent and with less responsibility.

Veterinary nurses currently play a role in preventative medicine. They frequently offer advice to clients on subjects ranging from parasite control to the management of a diabetic. They also administer medical treatment and perform minor surgery under the direction of the veterinary surgeon and in accordance with the Veterinary Surgeons Act and their Guide to Professional Conduct.

In 1992, The Veterinary Surgeons Act was amended and the role of the veterinary nurse was formally recognised in law in the Schedule Three amendment to the 1991 Act, a schedule that was amended again in 2002 (Appendix 2) to further increase the scope of the veterinary nurse's role.

There is no doubt that this amendment helped to increase recognition related to the role of the veterinary nurse and the training that veterinary nurses receive. However, some may argue that by defining what a veterinary nurse may or may not do in terms of medical treatment and minor surgery it continues to focus the veterinary nurse's role on the traditional medical model and gives fuel to the argument that veterinary nurses are, in fact, 'mini-vets'. This claim is strengthened by examining point 10 in the RCVS Guide to Professional Conduct for Veterinary Nurses 2004[10] (Appendix 1), which states that 'veterinary nurses should co-operate fully with veterinary surgeons assisting them in the provision of veterinary care'.

Although many veterinary nurses feel that the amendments made to Schedule Three of the Vet-

erinary Surgeons Act have placed restrictions on the tasks that they are able to perform, the role of the veterinary nurse has been constantly evolving and becoming more diverse. Over the past few years, veterinary nurses, in some practices, have started to perform tasks and take on responsibilities that back in 1961 would not have been considered. Nurse clinics are an example. In many practices, clients now make appointments to see veterinary nurses to discuss issues such as weight loss programmes and behavioural problems, a role that can be compared to that of a human 'nurse practitioner', one that was established within the National Health Service to improve patient education and enhance methods of preventative healthcare.[14]

Veterinary nurses need to examine their current role within practice, explore alternatives and formulate a definition of the role of a 'veterinary nurse'. Veterinary nurses could, of course, change their name to 'mini-vets,' maintaining a 'cure' focus to their work, or they could become professionals in their own right, by developing a role quite separate from that of a veterinary surgeon – one that has patient 'care' at its core and the interests of the animal at its heart. It could be argued that, as veterinary surgeons and veterinary nurses both currently utilise a 'cure' focus in their work, animal welfare is being compromised. Could the 'care' that patients and pet owners receive be improved?

THE CASE FOR RESEARCH

This question will only be answered if veterinary nurses carry out research and establish a body of knowledge specific to their role. It is widely believed that all professions need a knowledge base from which to practise. Indeed, one of the features attributed to a profession, is that it has a 'body of specific knowledge based on research'[15] which forms the basis for the decision making process. There is currently no body of knowledge available for veterinary nurses on which they can base their decisions and it is suggested that the care given to animals by veterinary nurses is currently based on:

- Tradition
- Belief

- Intuition
- Routine
- Trial and error

There is no doubt that experienced veterinary nurses have the ability to use clinical skills and past experiences to help them identify the care required by an individual patient but they currently do not have the research base to back up the decisions they make. In 2000, when referring to human nurses, McHaffie stated that 'good practice should be based wherever possible on sound evidence' and went on to say that it was 'not ethically acceptable to follow tradition or received wisdom without question'.[16]

In light of this evidence it could be argued that veterinary nursing is not a profession and it could be implied that veterinary nurses, by following tradition and not questioning the information that they receive are, in fact, not behaving in an ethical manner.

Hockey[17] identified a number of reasons why research was, and continues to be, needed within the field of human nursing. These reasons are relevant to the veterinary nurse:

Research has been described as 'an attempt to increase the sum of what is known, usually referred to as "a body of knowledge", by the discovery of new facts or relationships through a process of systematic scientific enquiry, the research process'.[17] In order for veterinary nursing to develop, it is imperative that within the next few years veterinary nursing research becomes part of the ethos of patient care.

IMPROVING PATIENT CARE: MOVING AWAY FROM A DISEASE FOCUS TO A PATIENT-FOCUSED APPROACH

This implies a move away from the 'medical model' to one that examines a patient not as an object but as an active subject with specific needs that may not be linked to the disease itself. It implies a change in attitudes towards working practice. It asks nurses to adopt a 'care focus' rather than a 'cure focus' and asks them to move away from performing tasks as a matter of routine, to thinking about the processes involved, and therefore involves problem-solving activities.

Assessment
This describes the process of history taking and patient observation. This is quite different from the history and observations that a veterinary surgeon will make, as it focuses on nursing care.

Box 1.2

1. To establish scientifically defensible reasons for nursing activities.
2. To provide nurses with an increased repertoire of scientifically defensible nursing intervention options.
3. To find ways of increasing the cost-effectiveness of nursing activities.
4. To provide a basis for standard setting and quality assurance.
5. To provide evidence of weaknesses and strengths in nursing.
6. To give the term evidence-based practice some credence.
7. To satisfy the academic curiosity of thinking nurses.
8. To facilitate interdisciplinary collaboration in nursing and nursing research.
9. To earn and defend a professional status for nursing.

Box 1.3   The nursing process

Faulkner, when referring to human nurses, described the nursing process as 'a method of nursing which concerns itself with an individual's physical, social and psychological reactions to disease, and which takes into account that the patient is a member of society with his own stresses within that society, which may affect his reaction to disease'.[18]

The process has four phases:

- Assessment
- Planning
- Implementation
- Evaluation

The veterinary nurse will ask the owner, for example, about the animal's daily routine and about its dietary requirements. The animal's behaviour will be examined once it is in the hospital ward. A general picture of the animal, its life and the owner will be established.

Planning
Correct assessment will help the veterinary nurse to identify actual and potential problems and, based on the evidence, make decisions relating to the care that is required and produce a plan of action.

Implementation
This is the 'caring' part of the process. The nurse needs to implement the care plan. The veterinary nurse should understand what is being done and have the skill to carry out the care. 'Many nursing actions could be carried out by the unskilled, but a skilled nurse is required to deliver a high standard of care.'[18]

Evaluation
This is a dynamic, ongoing process. If the nursing care being provided is not appropriate, it needs to be changed. Or the animal's needs may change, therefore a new approach needs to be taken. Assessment and evaluation are closely linked processes.

Veterinary nurses are beginning to challenge their role within the practice environment. The advent of veterinary nursing degree programmes and the redesigning of the diploma qualifications, together with the proposed changes in professional codes of conduct, policies and practice, demonstrate that veterinary nurses no longer wish to be thought of as 'hand maidens' to the veterinary surgeon but want to accept responsibility and operate from a position of professional accountability.

It is suggested that by moving away from the traditional nursing, medical model and implementing a nursing model that places the needs of the patient first, thereby developing a 'care focus,' veterinary nursing would become a unique, autonomous activity, quite separate from that of the veterinary surgeon.

If veterinary nurses are to become regulated, autonomous professionals, then further training and education are required in order for them to take on this responsibility effectively and efficiently. They will have to have an understanding of the processes involved and that will require a different kind of knowledge.

Education and training in the use of reflective practice is included in many of the degree programmes and therefore veterinary nurses qualifying via this route are already being introduced to this process. This does not mean that all veterinary nurses should undertake a degree programme but it may be time to evaluate and examine the training that is currently offered to certificate students to include more opportunities to evaluate and reflect on their practice.

Box 1.4   What is reflective practice?

Reflective practice has been around for a number of years and its links to effective learning have been well documented. It now forms part of VN degree programmes and student Veterinary Nurses are being encouraged to use it within their NVQ portfolios.

Reflection involves learners actively thinking about their past or current experiences. It includes the ability to be self-aware, to analyse experiences, to evaluate their meaning and to plan further action, therefore helping them to improve future performance.

The process of reflection
Various people have developed 'models' for the reflective process to help people to understand the concept. One model used has been devised by Atkins and Murphy[19] who describe the process as having four stages:

Stage 1 – Atkins and Murphy state that the process often starts with an awareness of uncomfortable feelings, usually due to new, unfamiliar, uncomfortable or negative situations. However this may not always be the case. There are occasions when reflecting on very positive situations will promote an understanding of how and why things worked out so well.

Stage 2 – This phase encourages the examination of the components of a situation, by breaking it down into simple parts and exploring alternative actions through research.

Stage 3 – This phase involves the collation of the facts and the production of a summary of the outcomes of reflection and learning.

Stage 4 – This phase involves the implementation of a plan of action resulting from the process of reflection.

The cycle is continuous as once the plan is implemented the new situation is reflected upon again.

CONCLUSION

It is up to veterinary nurses to drive this process of change forwards. It is time for nurses to be proactive and take responsibility for the direction that the profession is taking. This chapter has introduced the idea of the essential components for positive change, the five R's: regulation, responsibility, reflection, research and respect.

References

1. Turner T. Veterinary nursing: The first twenty five years. Harlow: British Veterinary Nursing Association; 1986.
2. Pitcher P. The first registered animal nursing auxiliary. In: Turner T. Veterinary nursing: the first twenty five years. Harlow: British Veterinary Nursing Association; 1986.
3. Earnshaw DG. The ethical aspects. In: Jones BV. Animal nursing, part 2. Oxford: Pergamon; 1966:282.
4. Ormrod AN. Medical nursing in relation to disease. In: Jones BV. Animal nursing, part 2. Oxford: Pergamon; 1966:417.
5. Turner J. Practical ethics for veterinary nurses. Veterinary practice nurse 1989; 1(4):22–23.
6. RCVS. VN responses to consultation paper. Online. Available: http://www.rcvs.org.uk/templates/internal.asp 8 May 2005.
7. Faulkner A. Nursing: a creative approach. London: Bailliere Tindall; 1985:428.
8. Johnston V. Some observations on animal nursing. Vet Rec 1962; 74(2):71.
9. Royal College of Nursing 2003. Defining nursing. Online. Available: http://www.rcn.org.uk/downloads/definingnursing/definingnursing-a5.pdf 9 May 2005.
10. RCVS Guide to Professional Conduct for Veterinary Nurses. In: RCVS List of Veterinary Nurses 2005: 193–194.
11. Younger JB. Themes in professional nursing practice. In: Creasia JL, Parker B, eds. Conceptual foundations: the bridge to professional nursing practice. 3rd edn. St Louis: Mosby; 2001:319–321.
12. Thompson IE, Melia KM, Boyd KM. Nursing ethics. 4th edn. Edinburgh: Churchill Livingstone; 2003.
13. Veterinary Surgeons Act 1966. London: HMSO.
14. Berry Z. Developing professions: nurse practitioners. Veterinary Nursing 2003; 18(5):152–154.
15. Burnard P, Chapman C. Professional and ethical issues in nursing. 3rd edn. Edinburgh: Bailliere Tindall; 2004:2.
16. McHaffie HE. Ethical issues in research. In: Cormack D, ed. The Research process in nursing. 4th edn. Oxford: Blackwell Science; 2000:52.
17. Hockey L. The nature and purpose of research. In: Cormack D, ed. The Research process in nursing. 4th edn. Oxford: Blackwell Science; 2000:4–7.
18. Faulkner A. Nursing: a creative approach. London: Bailliere Tindall; 1985:10–14.
19. Atkins S, Murphy K. Reflective practice. Nursing Standard 1994; 8(39):49–56.

Further reading

Wright B. Ethics in practice. Veterinary Practice Nurse 1994; 16(2):9–10.

2

Introduction to ethical principles

Siobhan Mullan

We all have to make decisions everyday about how to live our lives. Some of our decisions are straightforward matters of daily life that have no ethical dimension to them – for example, should I wear my red jumper or my green jumper today? On the other hand there are times when we have to make decisions based on our moral values – for example, should I tell my friend that her husband is having an affair? Ethics concerns the reasons *behind* our opinions on morally challenging questions. It goes beyond 'common practice', i.e. 'what people currently do' in a given situation, and encompasses notions such as 'good', 'bad', 'right' and 'wrong'. Although we will have made many ethical decisions during our lives, we may have been unaware of the type of reasoning behind our decisions. Knowledge of these reasons ensures a robust, logical and consistent approach to decisions we make in both our personal and professional lives. We will then be able to act in accordance with our values. This chapter will outline the main ethical theories used to consider moral problems and then offer some guiding principles of medical ethics and an ethical framework for decision-making in practice.

WHERE DO MORALS COME FROM?

Even before the ancient Greek philosophers, it is likely that people have considered ethical questions. This desire to make sense of how we decide what is right or wrong, fair or just, is very important, both to us as individuals and to society as a whole. It has been stated that 'morality serves two universal human needs. It regulates conflicts of interest between people, and it regulates conflicts of interest within the individual born of different desires and drives that cannot all be satisfied at the same time'.[1] It follows from this that morality is not optional as there will always be conflicts between and within us, that is, we are all moral agents. In order to be moral agents we need to be completely autonomous (a concept we will come back to with respect to our patients), i.e. we have complete moral freedom over our thoughts and actions and the ability for critical thinking. We recognise that people under extreme conditions (e.g. torture) are not able to think freely and we do not expect a baby (or an animal) to be a moral agent as they cannot reason. As a moral agent we have a responsibility to act morally both personally and at work where there is a specific expectation that we will behave conscientiously within our professional sphere. In addition, we must consider ethical issues critically and then *act* upon our reasoning. We must also be open to changing our views in response to reasoned arguments. Stirrat[2] has put forward some essential aspects of general and medical ethics:

- Ethics is for something and must be translatable into moral action. (It has to work in real life.)
- Each one of us is required to think ethically and act morally (i.e. we are all 'moral agents'.) (This is not an optional extra.)
- Ethics is about individuals living and working in a community. (It is not just about 'me' and 'mine'.)
- Individuals not only have rights but also duties/obligations towards others.
- The fundamental principles underpinning medical ethics are (or should be) those of society in general.

- We, as doctors [or veterinary surgeons or veterinary nurses] have special obligations or duties to our patients that are clearly laid down by the GMC [or RCVS].
- Clinical medicine, ethical analysis and moral action cannot be practised in isolation from one another. (Ethics is a necessary part of good clinical practice.)

WHO IS WORTHY OF MORAL CONSIDERATION?

Anything that is important *to us* will be considered in ethical questions. These have an *extrinsic value* and can include both animate objects, such as my friend, the animal I will eat or the bird I am enjoying watching, and inanimate objects such as my money or the environment I live in. In addition, we recognise that some things have their own *intrinsic* value. For example, we feel that people have their own worth that is important to themselves and requires protecting. This contrasts completely with how we view money – a coin has no value *to itself*. This intrinsic value demands a more complex consideration – and not just from the point of view of its usefulness to us. When we are considering differences in moral 'worth' we must make sure that we are concerning ourselves only with differences that are *morally relevant*. For example, we no longer consider skin colour a morally relevant difference between people and therefore discrimination on this basis is termed racism. Likewise, if we are to distinguish between humans and other animals in terms of the consideration we afford them, then there has to be a *morally relevant* difference between us, otherwise we would rightly be accused of *speciesism*. For example, if we are expecting to inflict pain on a person or an animal (as we might do in medical or veterinary practice) then the morally relevant issue would be the experience of pain felt by the subject. The term *sentience* is often linked to intrinsic value and encompasses notions such as the ability to think, feel pain and experience emotions. It is often considered a scale, with simple organisms at one end (a low level of sentience) and humans and other complex animals at the other end (a high level of sentience). Where on this scale we change

the moral weight we give to animals is a difficult decision. Should we afford the tapeworm the same protection as the cat?

HOW WILL I DECIDE WHAT TO DO?

There are two main ethical theories that usually guide our actions. In summary, these theories either involve an analysis of the likely costs (i.e. the harms done) and benefits, or they require that we always avoid certain harms or meet certain duties whatever the benefits. Although we may not be familiar with the history and philosophical thinking that underlies these theories, in practice we will be familiar with using these methods to make choices. Sometimes the same choice will result using either theory and sometimes very different choices will be made, depending upon which basis is used to make the decision.

How can I weigh everything up?

One possible way of considering ethical questions is to weigh up the costs and benefits of different courses of action – something we have probably all done without realising it. This is represented as a moral theory known as utilitarianism. An overview of utilitarianism can be encapsulated in the phrase 'the greatest good for the greatest number'. In a situation without a good outcome (a true ethical *dilemma*) the harm should be minimised – indeed we are familiar with the phrase 'choosing the lesser of two evils'. An important part of utilitarianism is that the expected consequences of any choice must be considered. It is therefore a *consequentialist* or *teleological* theory. There are several important points to note about utilitarianism briefly outlined below:

- We may not all agree on what is a harm and what is a benefit.

The early utilitarian Jeremy Bentham (1748–1832) considered 'happiness' to be limited to pleasurable experiences and the absence of pain. Refinements since then have included other, less immediate and hedonistic forms of happiness, for example the maintenance of one's dignity, or improving the structure of society. This 'happiness' is less

Table 2.1 The consequences of providing analgesia to animals

	Analgesic given	Analgesic not given
Animal consciously experiencing pain	✓ pain alleviated	✘ pain consciously experienced
Animal unable to consciously experience pain	✘ wasted resources	–

quantifiable than the straightforward pleasures in life and difficulties can arise in prioritising these. When considering animals in this light we need to be aware of their capabilities – mammals, birds, reptiles and fish can experience pleasures and pain (although there are still a few scientists who claim this is not *consciously* experienced). Utilitarianism can even be used to resolve this important issue practically. If we consider that we can never *know* whether an animal (or even another human being) is conscious we need to concern ourselves with the *consequences* of treating them as though they can or cannot feel meaningful pain. One useful way of doing this is to construct an ethical grid: (Table 2.1)

We can see that only the consequence of the action of providing analgesia to an animal that is feeling pain would result in 'happiness' (don't forget we are aiming for the goal of greatest happiness – positive pleasure or absence of pain) with the small potential cost of wasted time and expense if analgesia is actually not required. Conversely, if we look at the consequences of withholding analgesia from an animal consciously aware of pain then a large harm results from that animal being in pain. There is no harm or benefit to not providing analgesia to animals who are not feeling pain (this is sometimes termed a cost–neutral consequence). By this reasoning we *should* provide the analgesia.

The experience of pain for other animals is still being debated. It may also be that some animals do have a more complex awareness of 'happiness' in terms of an understanding of the future and the importance of social structure, which might need to be considered.

■ It can be very difficult to weigh up items that are not in the same 'currency'.

For example, on the same set of scales may be items such as pain, money, prolonged life, academic advancement, etc. In the example above we were weighing up the pain of an animal against the cost in time and money of providing analgesia. Changing circumstances may alter the values of costs and benefits. For example, if resources were scarce would it still be right to spend a large amount of money on alleviating pain for an animal, or if there were a more pressing demand on time – for example, in saving the life of another patient. Now the greatest good might be served by *not* providing analgesia.

■ It can be difficult to predict the outcome of our actions.

Research can sometimes improve our chances of estimating correctly. We can do this ourselves by using textbooks and journals, etc., but also as a society we are gaining more knowledge, which may be relevant in ethical issues. Again, looking at the example above, as a society we are learning more about the neurophysiology and behaviour related to the perception of pain that will inform us about the *likelihood* of the consequences of withholding analgesia. As practitioners we can then do our own research of the subject area, for example, to consider the likely requirement for, and consequences of, providing analgesia for a tarantula patient. The benefits in this case may not be so clear and the costs may include the potential harm caused by using untested drugs and unfamiliar techniques to administer the analgesic.

■ Individual 'rights' are barely considered.

As we have already said utilitarianism can be described neatly as 'the greatest good for the *greatest number'*. This 'majority rule' is an extremely important feature of this theory. Problems arise when the 'good' for an individual is at odds with the 'good' of a majority. For example, when the risk of a serious vaccination reaction becomes greater than the risk of the disease being vaccinated against, the *individual* would be best off not being vaccinated. However, if the *whole population* could be protected from the disease by *everyone* being vaccinated then the utilitarian would say that the 'good' of the majority should be served by vaccination.

Even more significantly, some of the individual rights that we might naturally take for granted can be disregarded if a greater good is served. For example, a utilitarian would argue that there is no such thing as a right to life and therefore it would be right to kill someone if not doing so would result in greater harm, such as the death of many more people.

- It may be skewed (or even abused by biased persons) by underestimation of costs and/or exaggeration of benefits.

As we have seen already, research will support the values we give to the costs and benefits. It is particularly important to be aware of unintentional bias in placing these values (especially in ourselves) and more particularly to consider the possibility of deception by others over the potential costs and benefits. For example, scientists may wish to conduct a piece of licensed research. They must present a detailed description of the *expected* costs to the animals and the benefits of this knowledge to society in order to gain a licence for the research. It would be possible to unintentionally (or even deliberately) underestimate the pain and other costs involved to the animal. If the scientists then also painted the best possible picture of the medical advances rather than a realistic expectation, the licence may be more likely to be granted, but using a flawed evaluation of the true situation.

Ultimately utilitarianism provides a very good tool for considering all the possible outcomes of an action and for resolving conflicts by making decisions that always result in achieving the goal of greatest 'happiness'.

Should I follow any rules?

Contrasting theories by which to make decisions concern making sure that we do the 'right' thing, rather than aiming for the most 'good' and are known as deontological theories. These theories assert that moral choices should be made following certain duties (rules) or in response to satisfying certain rights. These duties must be followed whatever the situation and in every similar situation, regardless of the consequences and regardless of whether this results in the greatest overall good. For example, we have a duty not to lie. Immanuel Kant (1724–1804) was an influential deontologist whose work is still discussed today. There are a number of important points to consider about deontology.

- The consequences of the action are irrelevant.

By ensuring that we abide by our duties, that in itself is 'right'. No consideration is made of anything that may result from following our duty. For example, if we consider that it is our duty not to lie, then we should not lie, even if we would be directing a murderer away from their intended victim by that lie. Deontological duties are often 'negative' constraints on our actions. In this case we could say instead that we have a duty to tell the truth, which is subtly different and harder to abide by.

- These theories are able to encompass the notion of individual 'rights'.

When we think of 'rights' we can mean many different things. With respect to animals it may simply mean that they are worthy of moral consideration. If we consider the provision of specific rights, we could say that a sheep has a right to graze grass – a sheep is *allowed* to graze grass. Further to that, we could say that a sheep has a right to defecate when she wants – *no-one may prevent* her from defecating at will. And even more stringently, we could say that a sheep has a right to a humane death – we have a *duty to provide* her with a humane death.

- Often these rights are enshrined in laws or professional codes.

By their nature, laws are identifiable rules defining our conduct. These tend to represent only the 'bottom-line' of acceptable behaviour and do not promote positive duties – 'we are bound only to comply with the letter of the law: we are not obliged to go beyond that and seek to embody its spirit in our deeds. If we can find loopholes in the law, we cannot be legally chastised if we choose to take advantage of them'.[3] If we take our example of our duty not to lie, we can see that, because of the narrow nature of this duty, in a court of law this has been transformed into telling 'the truth, the whole truth and nothing but the truth' in order to avoid loopholes. Codes of conduct, by contrast, are often able to outline positive duties expected of us.

- Choosing a rule that is applicable in every situation can be very difficult.

When considering a deontological rule, it is important that the rule must be followed in every similar situation. One way of thinking about this is to consider what would happen if everybody was to follow this rule. Let's consider again the rule not to lie. Even if we wanted to tell a small lie, by this reasoning it would be wrong, because if everybody lied when they wanted to, we would never know when anyone was telling the truth, and the whole structure of society would be undermined. Some deontologists, however, recognise the difficulty of the rigid application of the rules, and allow exceptions to be made for extreme circumstances.

- Rules, duties or rights may conflict with each other.

What happens when my right to treat my pet as I wish conflicts with their right to avoid suffering – such as the pain and distress associated with neutering? In such cases we need to be able to prioritise our rules. This could be done on the basis of avoiding the worst harms, avoiding harming the worst off or choosing to harm the fewest number of individuals. This problem can become apparent at work – who do we have a primary duty towards, our patients, our employer or the client?

In summary, deontology is particularly useful for its ability to safeguard the interests of the individual. This may be particularly important for vulnerable members of our society and animals.

What do we do as a society?

In practice, a combination of these theories can be used. For example, both theories are encompassed in the legislation covering the use of animals for scientific procedures. Licence applications are judged on a cost–benefit analysis (utilitarianism). In this the costs to the animals (e.g. pain/ confinement, etc.) are weighed up against the expected benefit to humans (e.g. new medications/ knowledge, etc.). However, the government has also decreed, for example, that no licences will be granted for procedures on great apes (deontology), regardless of any potential benefits. In fact, a combination of theories is often used in social ethics, as Rollin [4] has stated:

> Although we make most of our social decisions by considering what will produce the greatest benefit for the greatest number, a utilitarian/teleological/consequentialist ethical approach, we skilfully avoid the 'tyranny of the majority' or the submersion of the individual under the weight of the general good. We do this by considering that the individual is, in some sense, inviolable. Specifically, we consider those traits of an individual that we believe are constitutive of his or her *human nature* to be worth protecting at almost all costs.

IS THERE ANYTHING ELSE THAT CAN HELP ME?

There are some other concepts are particularly relevant to us as professionals involved in veterinary health care. They may be useful to consider when contemplating our difficult ethical cases.

What do doctors do?

Medical ethics have developed the main ethical theories into four general principles to guide our actions.[5] For veterinary surgeons and veterinary nurses these principles apply primarily to actions affecting the animals that we are involved with, as enshrined in the veterinary oath: 'I . . . further promise that . . . my constant endeavour will be to ensure the welfare of animals committed to my care.'

1. Non-maleficence. This is the principle of not doing harm. It is often thought of as the first principle to follow – whatever we do we mustn't make things worse. However, veterinary practice often inflicts short term harm on animals that must be weighed up against the long term good expected. This is also taken into account in animal cruelty legislation where to cause an animal 'suffering' can be permissible in cases where it is deemed 'necessary' – for example, the suffering associated with a simple fracture repair.

2. Beneficence. This principle of promoting good follows once non-maleficence is ensured. In this respect we should try to improve the welfare of animals under our care in the short term and long term wherever possible. Beneficence is often combined with non-maleficence in order to determine the 'best interest' of an animal.

3. Autonomy. Autonomy relates to the ability of people or animals to be self-governing. The bottom line for respecting autonomy usually ends when laws are broken, but professional codes and acting as a moral agent are also important. Conflicts can arise between two autonomous people, for example, veterinary surgeon and client. Respecting animal autonomy might involve allowing them to make certain choices about their life (e.g. when to eat/sleep, etc.).

4. Justice. Justice can be thought of as treating all animals and all people in a fair and equal way. This can be thought of in many different ways. For example, if we have a finite set of resources we could divide them equally between everyone (or every animal). Perhaps a more appropriate way of dealing with health care resources is to divide them up according to need. For example, we should consider the *needs* of all animals equally and be aware that these needs will differ for each individual, even within the same species.

How should I be?

If we are the type of person who is, for example, caring by nature, then it is likely that we will carry out caring acts. Virtue ethics maintains that it is *how we are* that is important and that if we are a 'virtuous' or 'morally good' person then we will naturally act correctly in accordance with our character. Virtue ethics can be used in conjunction with theories of ethical reasoning, and returning to this central question of how I should be can be especially useful when considering what is expected of us as a professional. There are certainly particular characteristics, for example, compassion, honesty and fairness that we, as health care workers, are especially expected to possess.

Can other views also be right?

Once we have completed our moral reasoning in a particular case and come to our answer we might wonder whether it is the *only* right answer. In other words is there a single moral truth? Ethical relativism would say that every moral issue is necessarily and relevantly framed within an individual, cultural or social context. In its most extreme form, it is logically indefensible, as it is impossible to pass judgement on other people's views or try to convert them to your own. In a more tempered form it can be useful within the medical professions to guard against the 'doctor knows best' attitude, which we are now shifting away from. This paternalistic approach did not necessarily take into account other people's (patients/clients) views and certainly did not assume them to be as valid as one's own.

A PRACTICAL FRAMEWORK FOR MAKING ETHICAL DECISIONS

Sometimes we can get lost amongst all the information surrounding an ethical issue. A framework for making decisions can ensure that we do not fail to consider any important points. This is the framework that I use in practice.

1. Identify all the possible courses of action.
2. Establish the interests of affected parties, including any related legal or professional guidance.

3. Formulate an ethical decision.
4. Minimise the impact of the decision.

Identify possible courses of action

At the presentation of a case it is important to consider all the possible options. At this point it is important that this is done comprehensively, as it is impossible to evaluate something that has not been considered. This process must be an assessment of the possible courses of action free of personal opinions/values. Values can be imposed later in order to decide which options have merit. In many cases the potential options will include taking no action or euthanasing the animal, in addition to various treatment options. In other cases options might also include palliative treatment or further diagnostic investigations – all either at the practice or a referral institution.

Consideration of all interested parties

Understanding the interests of parties involved in ethical decision-making can help to outline the reasons for holding a particular view on treatment options. In order to engage in a discussion, these underlying motives can then be considered as to whether they are reasonable and should be influencing any decision. The immediate parties usually involved will be the animal, its owner and the veterinary surgeon/ nurse. A consideration of the animal's welfare is obviously paramount. It can be useful to use established principles of animal welfare in order to ensure that all aspects are considered, for example, the 'Five Freedoms'. In addition, the severity, duration and numbers of animals affected by any ethical decisions may need to be taken into account.

Conflicts between interested parties are often central to ethical problems. For example:

- Should a client request euthanasia of an incontinent animal because they have visitors arriving?
- Should a nurse assist in a procedure she is unhappy with because her employer has told her to?
- Should a veterinary surgeon encourage bringing forward an inevitable euthanasia to a more convenient time for him/herself?

- Should a farmer be allowed to refuse pain-relieving treatment on economical grounds?

The motives underlying some of these questions may not always be 'good' or 'appropriate' so it is important to be aware of all factors that influence people's actions, in order to guard against making inappropriate choices.

In addition to considering the interests of the parties immediately involved, a wider approach can be taken by looking at the views of society and professional bodies, as encompassed in the law and professional guidance respectively. This means that options that result in a law or a professional code being broken will be discounted at an early stage. Since the various justifications vary, the law or guidelines may differ between each species; for example, tail docking is legally prohibited in cattle and horses, but is allowed, subject to certain legal restrictions, in pigs, sheep and dogs. However, the RCVS considers tail docking in dogs to be an 'unjustified mutilation'.

Formulating an ethical decision

There are two parts to this step:

Identifying the ethical issues involved
In many theoretical examples the ethical decisions required are neatly outlined. However, in real life cases, teasing out the ethical issues central to the problem can be very difficult. Sometimes information that is put persuasively, or with force, can take on a significance that it does not warrant, thereby obscuring the real underlying issue. Central to all veterinary ethical decisions will be a consideration of any rights we believe the animal to have, or a consideration of the animal welfare compromises likely to result from any decision made.

Choosing a course of action
This is where the hard work really begins! All the above information needs to be condensed into whichever ethical principles you personally subscribe to. It may be that you wish to perform a utilitarian cost/ benefit analysis or it may be that you believe you have certain deontological duties to carry out or that some of the affected parties have specific rights to be considered. You may be required to prioritise your deontological rules.

Physically writing down these rules, or items to be balanced along with a grid of the interests of the affected parties, can be helpful. This is also the point to consider our extra tools to help us – what would happen if I followed the four principles of medical ethics? How should I be in this situation? And finally, can I accept that someone else's opposing views may also be right?

Minimising the impact of ethical decisions

Once a decision has been made a consideration of how to further minimise harm must be undertaken. This final step is often termed 'refinement', where it limits the impact on the individual animal. This is a part of the decision-making process that is easily overlooked, however, it is an important way of reducing the impact of that decision. Examples of refinement could include:

- An improved analgesic regimen.
- Use of environmental enrichment.
- Attending to psychological/ emotional needs of the patient.
- Choosing a drug with fewer side effects.
- Protecting against expected adverse effects.
- Restricting numbers of animals affected.

SOME REAL-LIFE CASE EXAMPLES

We will look at each of the following four cases in a particular light to demonstrate how the principles we have been discussing apply to real life cases.

Box 2.1 Renal transplantation in cats

A client wishes to discuss the possibility of referral for renal transplantation for her three-year-old Persian cat with polycystic kidney disease (PKD). Your practice principal has made it clear that she is totally against the procedure. A local hospital has already carried out several renal transplants in cats. They will not see any clients without a referral letter from the original practice. The client has asked to speak to you as the head nurse. What are *your* views on renal transplantation?

Guiding principles of medical ethics:

Non-maleficence: For your client's cat there will certainly be a short term harm associated with the surgical procedure and some longer term harms from the extensive follow-up care required. The question arises of whether you need to consider the harm done to the source cat by removing its kidney. Although that cat is not your client, as a veterinary professional you probably need to concern yourself with all the animals that might be affected by your decisions.

Beneficence: The aim is to increase the length of life for your client's cat – certainly a beneficent cause. Of course, it is not clear that this would necessarily be the case. The disease progression of PKD is variable and there could be problems associated with the transplant. When considering the source cat it is hard to see how the procedure could be considered beneficent. Depending upon the circumstances of the source cat it may be guaranteed a home (if it was a stray) with the recipient's family as part of the bargain. This could be very positive, although there could still be concerns regarding whether it would be socially compatible with the recipient cat or whether it would be cared for equally.

Autonomy: The ability of the recipient cat to be self-determining may well be reduced, when compared with a healthy cat, during the perioperative period and by the frequent follow-up treatments required following transplantation. However, the autonomy of a sick animal is very poor and therefore without the transplant this may be more compromised. There are two ways of considering the autonomy of the source cat. Firstly, you might consider that, once recovered, the cat is clinically healthy, and is able to live its life exactly as autonomously as if it had two kidneys – at least up until such a point as that one remaining kidney began to function less well. On the other hand, you may consider that actually autonomy goes further than that, and therefore it is not possible for autonomy to be respected by removing fundamental parts of a body.

Justice: Now you have to consider how to treat these cats in a fair way. As we have said already, there can be several ways to consider this. Firstly, dividing up resources equally by providing a kidney transplant to all cats would be ridiculous. This is a case that must be judged by *need*. Here we have a cat that needs a transplant but we also have a cat who has little interest in giving away a kidney. Are we considering both of their positions fairly? Would the client be willing to use another of their cats as a source for the kidney? Utilitarian justice would say that the fairest way of considering this would be to produce the greatest overall good. In the stark terms of overall length of life produced by this procedure (the sum of the lifespan of the source and recipient cats) then performing the transplant would be fairest. At this point we should note that in medical ethics we only include items such as time and money when considering the resources to be divided up. We do not consider that the kidneys themselves can be divided up on a needs basis – otherwise we would all be compulsorily tissue typed, registered and required to donate a kidney if needed. You should consider whether there are any *morally relevant* differences between the human and feline situations.

CONCLUSION

When considering both cats, there are many harms, with some benefits, to transplantation. Autonomy will not be promoted and there appears to be no morally relevant differences between cats and humans that would allow us to go against the social ethic of not requiring body parts to be divided up amongst the population fairly. Using the guiding principles of medical ethics, you cannot support kidney transplantation in cats as it currently exists, and should explain this to your client.

Box 2.2 Feeding a vegetarian dog

A new client brings in a retired greyhound that they have recently acquired and asks the nurse for advice on diet and health care. They tell the nurse that they plan to feed the dog a commercially prepared vegetarian dog food. The nurse tells them it is unfair to force their dog to be vegetarian. What would you do?

We are going to consider this situation using virtue ethics and relativism. Firstly, let's assume that although it is not 'natural' and there are some potential health concerns, it is possible to provide adequate nutrition for a vegetarian dog.

Virtue ethics: How should I be in this situation? Clearly we are expected to be compassionate, caring and truthful individuals, with integrity in the way we are to both animals and people. If you are true to these virtues, then you will convey what you believe to be in the best interests of the dog. You won't try to put emotional pressure on the owners, but you will discuss with them your reasons why you believe a meat diet to be better. Clearly, they will see from this that your main interest is in the welfare of their dog and not in any other less virtuous reasons, such as wanting to sell them your pet food. However, you have to acknowledge that this is not a major issue, as it is possible to maintain a healthy dog on a vegetarian diet. You also respect the owners and when they still resist the meat option, you advise them on how to ensure good health for their dog on a vegetarian diet.

Relativism: You feel strongly that some meat is best for dogs and you think it is wrong to do anything that might be harmful to a dog. If you are also a relativist, then you can accept that your clients have a different view. They are more concerned with the poor welfare of 'factory farmed' animals and do not want to be a part of that system – a view you have some sympathy with. You are able to discuss your concerns with them and agree to differ on the fundamental underlying issues. You are also able to advise them on where to get 'welfare friendly' meat and a good vegetarian diet.

Box 2.3 A personal ethical dilemma

An owner brings in a heavily pregnant cat and informs the veterinary surgeon that she cannot cope with a litter of kittens. The veterinary surgeon estimates the pregnancy to be at the seven-week stage. The owner wishes to have the cat spayed, otherwise she will have to take her to a cat rescue shelter. The veterinary surgeon agrees to carry out the operation. The theatre nurse does not wish to be involved as she has strong views on terminating pregnancies. Should she agree to assist?

We will consider this dilemma from a deontological, 'duties' perspective.

Deontology: The nurse clearly feels strongly that termination of a pregnancy is wrong. This is a 'deontological constraint' for her, which she must not go against. She therefore has a duty not to be a part of this surgical procedure that would necessarily result in the deaths of the kittens. As no consideration is taken of the consequences of her actions, she must still avoid violating her deontological constraint by refusing to assist, even if it meant that an inexperienced trainee would be required to help instead. She also has no obligation to go against her rule just because it would mean that someone else would be put in the same position. In this case she has a conflict of duties as she also has a duty to her employer – both morally and legally, in the form of an employment contract. She did not tell her employer before she started work that she held these beliefs. In this case, she needs to find a satisfactory way of prioritising the harms committed by not fulfilling one of the duties. If she agrees to assist then she will have committed a harm concerning life and death – an important matter. On the other hand, if she does not agree then she has failed in her obligations towards her employer – a less serious harm – and so this is what she could do.

Box 2.4 Injection of methyl-prednisolone into the fetlock joints of a horse

You have been asked to assist with the administration of methyl-prednisolone into all four fetlock joints of a three-day eventer the day before it is due to compete. The veterinary surgeon asks that on this occasion you do not clip the hair around the injection site. The client is a well-known rider with a number of horses. You have concerns with assisting with this procedure because you know the horse is going to be more prone to serious injury and chronic damage, and you are asked to ignore the practice policy for surgical skin preparation, making you suspicious that it is not all 'above board'. Do you agree to assist?

We will now use our ethical framework to discuss this case.

1. Identify all the possible courses of action. You can either agree to assist or refuse to assist, with or without reporting to the sport's governing body if appropriate.
2. Establish the interests of affected parties.
   - *Horse*: The horse has some mild osteo-arthritic changes in the fetlock joints, which at present do not appear to be very painful although may have some detrimental effect during hard competition. The horse has an interest in avoiding pain and distress and in its long-term health and welfare.
   - *Owner*: They want the horse to be as fit as possible for this event and possibly for future events. They are probably concerned to some degree about the welfare of the horse and not breaking any rules governing doping in their sport. However, by presenting the horse for the treatment they have shown that this is not their primary concern.
   - *Veterinary surgeon*: They should want to promote the welfare of the horse as a priority. They will also be concerned with complying with owners' wishes, maintaining the high view of the profession in the eyes

of the public and acting within the RCVS guidelines. They may also be concerned to keep a profitable client.

- *British Eventing*: This governing body has an interest in fair competition and the welfare of the horses taking part in the sport. If there was a welfare or doping problem it may affect the public perception of the sport. Their rules governing prohibited substances in horses state that 'substances capable at any time of acting on . . . the musculoskeletal system' and 'analgesics and anti-inflammatory substances' are prohibited.[6]
- *Spectators/ society*: The people enjoying watching the sport want to see a fair competition between horses. Although there are many who would be disappointed if a particular horse was not present, they are likely to respect a decision to withdraw due to lameness, as they would be concerned for the animal's welfare.

3. Formulate an ethical decision. As this is clearly against the rules of the sport's governing body, this is your first concern and as you do not wish to be a part of a doping offence you are not willing to assist. However, you suspect that this practice is widespread and wish to consider the implications further – clearly the veterinary surgeon you work for, whom you have a great deal of respect for, is happy to carry this out. If you do not agree to assist it is likely to be carried out anyway – unless you are able to persuade the veterinary surgeon and owner by your reasoning – or possibly threaten to report the incident to the governing body. You consider a utilitarian evaluation to be most useful in this case. (Table 2.2)

When you examine the case further you see that if you are not going to report the incident then the risks to the horse and the veterinary surgeon need to weighed up against the strength of your principles against doping in sport. Everything else is unaffected, as the procedure would go ahead anyway. Although you feel some obligation towards both the horse and the veterinary surgeon you feel that it is more important to abide by the rules – particularly as it does not appear to be in the long-term interest of the horse anyway. Your final option of threatening to report the incident may help the horse the most, if your threat is successful, as it could prevent this treatment. On the other hand, if it is not able to compete at the level required, its welfare cannot be assumed to be preserved as presumably it would not be of much use for its present owner. If the injections still go ahead and you report the incident to the governing body then you will set in motion a huge chain of events that could have far reaching consequences – both for people that you know and also many others, such as sponsors of the sport. However, you may be able to prevent further cases of doping, thereby promoting the welfare of other horses. Luckily, this time, by reasoning with the veterinary surgeon and owner you are able to persuade them not to perform the injections.

4. Minimise the impact of the decision. You are able to direct the owner to an equine physiotherapist who applied legitimate treatments to the horse prior to the competition.

Table 2.2 Consequences of possible actions

	Agree to assist (procedure will to go ahead)	Do not agree to assist (procedure likely to go ahead)	Consequences of reporting incident
Horse	?Short term pain relief. Small risk of joint sepsis due to inadequate preparation.	?Short term pain relief. Greater risk of joint sepsis due to inadequate preparation and lack of assistance.	If just threatening is successful at preventing injections: prevention of long-term hastening of joint disease and therefore pain. May end sporting career.
Owner	May get better placing in competition.	May get better placing in competition.	Possible disqualification from the sport.
Veterinary surgeon	Receives money. Helps client. Safe procedure.	Receives money. Helps client. At risk from kicking.	Possible disciplinary hearing.
Spectators/ society	Will see a favourite horse – possibly winning. Will be watching an unfair competition.	Will see a favourite horse – possibly win. Will be watching an unfair competition.	Will be aware of doping issues and may lose confidence in the sport – especially if there are more cases.
British Eventing	Will be hosting an unfair event. May be interested in selection for international competitions that may now be skewed.	Will be hosting an unfair event. May be interested in selection for international competitions that may now be skewed.	Possible loss of sponsors for the sport. May prevent further doping incidences.
Nurse (You!)	Go against your principles.	Allow more risk to horse and veterinary surgeon by not having an assistant.	May lose your job. Will have to appear before disciplinary hearing against veterinary surgeon and owner and may be cross examined.

References

1. Wong D. Relativism. In: Singer P, ed. A companion to ethics. Oxford: Blackwell; 1993.
2. Stirrat GM. How to approach ethical issues: a brief guide. The Obstetrician & Gynaecologist 2003; 5:130–135.
3. Davis NA. Contemporary deontology. In: Singer P, ed. A companion to ethics. Oxford: Blackwell; 1993.
4. Rollin BE. An introduction to veterinary medical ethics: theory and cases. Ames: Iowa State University Press; 1999:27.
5. Beauchamp TL , Childress JF. Principles of biomedical ethics. 4th edn. Oxford: Oxford University Press; 1994.
6. International Federation for Equestrian Sports. FEI list of prohibited substances July 2004. Online. Available: http://62.2.231.126 11 May 2005.

Further Reading

Mullan SM, Main DCJ. Principles of ethical decision-making in veterinary practice. In Practice 2001; 23(7):394–401.
Walsh P. VN's and the law: what would you do? Veterinary Nursing 2003; 18(4):117–120.

3

Introduction to the legal system

Carol Gray and Kathryn Wilson

INTRODUCTION

Any textbook which tries to describe law and the law-making process runs the risk of becoming bogged down in legal terminology, with a dry list of cases and procedures. In this chapter we have tried to concentrate on the essential information for any student of ethics and law. We will examine the legal system, how legislation is made and updated, the main differences between criminal and civil law and the meaning of accountability in law.

It is impossible to develop a set of ethical principles without some knowledge of the legal boundaries which apply. The law provides a set of written rules and sets precedents for dealing with similar situations in the future. However, something that you consider to be morally wrong may in fact be legally permissible. It is up to each individual to develop an ethical code, which may go a stage further than the relevant legislation.

WHAT IS LAW?

It is very difficult to find a written definition of law. According to Sir John Salmond 'law is the body of principles recognised and applied by the state in the administration of justice'.[1] Law is concerned with providing a just system of punishment, and providing a system for redress, against wrongdoing. (Fig. 3.1)

CRIMINAL LAW

Criminal law is concerned with the punishment of offences by the State, in order to protect society and individuals from harm. It tends not to get involved where there is a dispute between two parties with little risk of harm to either of them, or to any others. The Crown (via the Crown Prosecution Service) brings prosecutions against defendants (the people accused of committing a crime). Prosecutions are rarely instigated by individuals (private prosecutions) or by other organisations (e.g., the RSPCA, which is still responsible for prosecuting cases under the Protection of Animals Act 1911). There are three types of criminal offence:

- Summary – relatively minor offences, but includes animal cruelty cases. These cases are tried in Magistrates Courts, where evidence is heard by magistrates, who decide on the defendant's guilt and sentence/fine.
- Indictable – more serious offences such as murder and rape. These are tried in the Crown Court in front of a judge and jury. The jury decides on the defendant's guilt, and the judge decides on sentence.
- Triable either way – the offence falls between the two categories above, and the defendant can elect for a trial by jury rather than magistrates. This category includes burglary and robbery.

Most crimes are defined by statute (Acts of Parliament), although the crime of murder is a notable exception. This is still dependent on common law, unwritten law that is handed down through previous judgments in similar cases. Sentences for murder are, however, defined by statute.

Scots criminal law

Scotland also has a system of prosecution by a public prosecutor. In the lower Court, any criminal

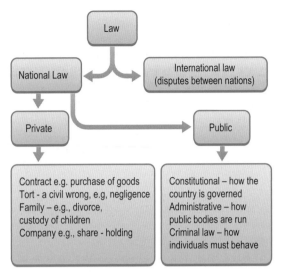

Figure 3.1 **Types of law.**

prosecutions are in the name of the Procurator Fiscal, and in the High Court, prosecutions are in the name of the Lord Advocate. Under Scots Law, cases are brought either in the District Court, before a Justice of the Peace or a Stipendiary Magistrate (covering minor offences including road traffic offences), in the Sheriff Court, before a Sheriff or Sheriff and jury, and before a Judge and jury in the High Court of Justiciary. Under Scots Law, it is not possible to elect for trial by jury in a Criminal case. Serious prosecutions such as murder, rape, etc., are commenced by way of Indictment and are prosecuted in the High Court which is also the final Court of Appeal in criminal cases.

Any appeal against refusal of bail, conviction and/or sentence in the Sheriff Court, is brought before the High Court, as the final Court of Appeal in criminal matters. Cases can also be referred to the High Court of Appeal by the Scottish Criminal Case Review.

It is still possible, although extremely rare, for a private prosecution to be brought. The procedure for this is by way of a bill of criminal letters, and the party wishing to proceed applies to the Lord Advocate for his concurrence in the bill. It is also possible, although rare, for prosecutions to be brought by public bodies (for example, Customs & Excise), or under the Education Act, but these are brought by the Procurator Fiscal rather than the

public body. The Scottish system is an accusatorial system which means that the Procurator presents the relevant evidence, rather than the judge investigating the same.

CIVIL LAW

Civil law is concerned with harm or loss suffered by an individual, either as a result of a crime or a failure to fulfil obligations towards another person. An example of a crime that results in a civil action is a case of dangerous driving, resulting in serious injury to a pedestrian or another driver.

However, more commonly, civil actions result from a breach of 'duty of care', owed by every individual and organisation to everyone else.

A 'tort' is a wrong against someone's personal safety, possessions or reputation. In veterinary practices, the most common civil actions are breach of contract, trespass and negligence. For example, negligence causes injury via breach of duty of care (e.g. by allowing an animal to injure a client). Trespass involves interference with someone's property (including animals; for example, the performance of an unauthorised surgical procedure). Breach of contract means that the terms of a contract (e.g. for veterinary treatment) have not been fulfilled (for example, a surgical procedure has not been carried out).

Decisions in civil cases are usually financial (compensation, damages) or prohibitive (known as an injunction, which, for example, can prevent someone from continuing with some work, or from having contact with another individual).

Civil law in Scotland

The Scottish legal system has no concept of tort. Instead, wrongs, or breaches of a legal duty to individuals which cause unjustifiable harm, are dealt with under the law of delict. This includes work-related claims for damages, injuries caused by road traffic accidents, nuisance claims and professional negligence claims. In Scotland, an injunction is known as an interdict.

Cases covered by the laws of delict or contract are litigated in the Sheriff Court before a Sheriff, or can be brought and indeed, in certain situations, must be brought before the Court of Session. Under Scots Law, the only time an individual can elect for trial by jury is in a civil action at the Court of Session. Cases brought in the Court of Session tend to be for larger sums of money or involve more complex areas of law.

Any appeal from a decision by a Sheriff in civil matters can proceed to the Sheriff Principal or the Inner House of the Court of Session sitting as an Appeal Court.

In Scots Law, cases of a very low monetary value, i.e. Small Claims (under £750) or Summary Causes (claims valued from £750 to £1,500), are dealt with by a Sheriff, and an appeal against a decision on a point of law is brought before the Sheriff Principal. There is no appeal to the Court of Session in a Small Claim.

If an individual has appealed to the Sheriff Principal and subsequently to the Inner House of the Court of Session sitting as an Appeal Court, but is still aggrieved by the decision, then they can appeal to the House of Lords sitting as an appellant Court.

Box 3.1

An individual living in Berwick upon Tweed, who uses a veterinary practice across the border in Scotland, is dissatisfied with the veterinary surgeon's treatment of their dog. The veterinary surgeon administered an antiparasitic drug which killed their valuable pedigree Border Collie. The client would be required to raise an action against the veterinary surgeon in Scotland, either on the basis of the veterinary surgeon's place of business, or the place of performance of the delict (i.e. the action leading to the damages claim). If dissatisfied with the decision of the local Sheriff Court, then an appeal against that decision would be made to either the Sheriff Principal or the Inner House of the Court of Session in Edinburgh. If still unhappy with the decision (which presumably has been that the veterinary surgeon has not been negligent), then the very rich individual would be entitled to appeal against this decision to the House of Lords in London, thus bringing the matter back into England, albeit by way of the Scottish Court system! (Table 3.1)

HOW LEGISLATION IS MADE

Law originates from legislation, written as Acts of Parliament, and from 'precedent' arising from judicial decisions in previous, similar cases. Increasingly, UK law is influenced by law originating from the European Union. Some of this law will require a change in UK law, while some is directly applicable. Cases decided in British courts may be overturned in the European Court. Decisions taken by the higher courts are binding on all lower courts.

Statutes are developed from Bills presented to both Houses of Parliament. Bills are usually sponsored by the Government but may also be presented by an individual MP – a Private Member's Bill. Government-sponsored Bills are allotted more parliamentary time than Private Members' Bills and these consequentially have less chance of becoming law unless they also have Government support. This happened with the bid to ban hunting. Several Private Members' Bills to ban hunting were introduced over a period of time, without success, until eventually the Labour Party included this in their manifesto.[2] (Fig. 3.2)

More recent statutes often provide a broad legislative framework and allow ministers to produce detailed regulations for the operation of the law. The original statute is known as an Enabling Act, and the regulations derived from it are known as Statutory Instruments. Around 2000 Statutory Instruments are produced from government departments each year. This type of legislation is known as delegated legislation and is a more flexible method of changing the law.

At any voting stage in the House of Commons, a Bill can be thrown out and will then have to start the process again, probably running out of time in a particular Parliamentary session. In the House of Lords any proposed amendments, or total rejection, mean that the Bill must go back to the Third Reading stage in the House of Commons. Under the Parliament Act, the House of Lords cannot reject a Bill more than twice. This was the case with the Hunting Act 2004.[3]

The Scottish legislative process

In 1998, the Scotland Act[4] brought into being a new layer of government for Scotland by way of a

Table 3.1   The differences between Criminal and Civil Law in England

Question	Criminal	Civil
What is the purpose of this type of law?	To maintain law and order to protect.	To uphold the rights of the individual.
What is the purpose of the trial?	To decide the defendant's guilt.	To decide if there has been a breach of these rights.
Who starts the case?	The State (the police or Crown Prosecution Service). In English law a private prosecution can be brought by an individual or an organisation, e.g. RSPCA.	The individual whose rights have been affected.
What is the legal term for that person?	Prosecutor.	Plaintiff.
Where are the cases heard?	Magistrates Court and Crown Court.	County Court and High Court.
Who decides?	Magistrates, jury.	Judge, rarely jury.
What is the decision?	Guilty/not guilty.	Liable/not liable.
What are the powers of redress?	Prison, fine, probation.	Damages, injunction, etc.
How is the case identified?	R v. defendant (R = Regina (the Crown), v. = Versus, defendant = defendant's surname).	Gray v. Pullen.
What type of proof is required?	Beyond reasonable doubt.	On the balance of probabilities.

directly elected parliament, and on May 6 1999 voting took place for the first Scottish Members of Parliament known as MSPs. The Scotland Act allows the Scottish Parliament to legislate on devolved issues. There are, however, many matters that are still reserved to the UK Parliament, one of these being the regulation of the veterinary profession.

Since the Scottish Parliament's inception, it has passed a number of ground-breaking Acts, such as the Protection of Wild Mammals (Scotland) Act 2002[5], which banned hunting in Scotland, prior to the English Act.

In December 2004, historic judgment was delivered at Jedburgh Sheriff Court in the case of the Procurator Fiscal Jedburgh against Trevor Adams.[6] This was the first prosecution to be brought under the Protection of Wild Mammals Act. It was held that the activity which had been undertaken by the accused was flushing foxes from cover above ground, that the accused was searching for foxes for the purpose of flushing them from cover in order that they might be shot, and that the dogs were under control at the time. The accused's activities accordingly fell within the terms of Section 2(2) of the Act and he was not guilty of the offence. Interestingly, it has been suggested that the accused would have been found guilty under the English legislation.[7]

There are differences between Westminster and Holyrood, the Scottish Parliament, the main differences being:

■ at Holyrood there is no second chamber (House of Lords),
■ any Act raised by the Scottish Parliament must be within legislative competence (i.e. what the Scottish Parliament is allowed to legislate for),
■ the Member in charge of the bill, i.e. the Minister introducing the bill, and the Presiding Officer must make statements that the bill is within the legislative competence,
■ the Law Officers and the Secretary of State for Scotland have power to refer any bill to the

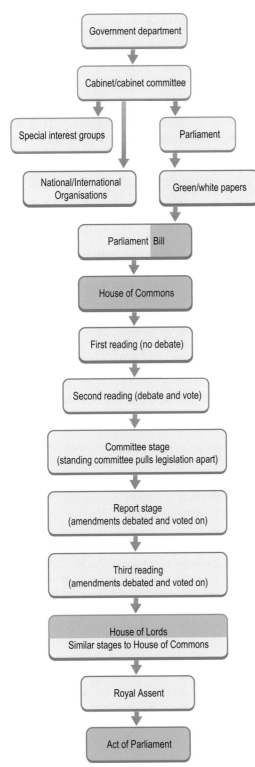

Figure 3.2 **How does a Bill become law?**

Judicial Committee of the Privy Council for a decision as to its 'vires,' i.e. its competence. This prohibits the bill's progress to Royal Assent.

The majority of the bills which are introduced at Holyrood are executive bills, which are the same as Government-sponsored bills. The Scottish Parliament also has Members' Bills which are the same as Private Members' Bills.

HOW THE LAW IS CHANGED

Parliament is directly responsible for most of the new legislation that is introduced each year. How can a member of the public, or a profession, influence this process?

Laws are changed for several reasons:

Government policy.
Each party outlines its proposals for new legislation in its pre-election manifesto
Changing values in society.
Moral issues can produce a change in public opinion, which is picked up by MPs. Pressure groups can lobby MPs to try to get a change in the government's policy.

Technological advances

New technologies or inventions may require new legislation or a change to existing legislation.

Law reform

The Law Commission carries out regular reviews of existing legislation and proposes any reforms it feels are necessary. If the government feels that a particular area is in need of a review, it may select a special committee to carry this out.

European legislation

New legislation, or a change to existing legislation, may be required to bring the UK into line with the European Union. NB some EU laws are directly applicable without recourse to the UK legislative process. (Fig. 3.3)

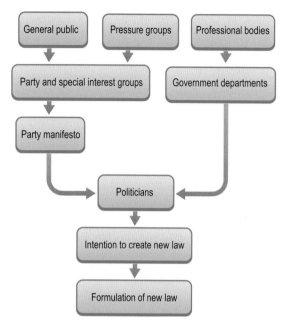

Figure 3.3 **Diagram highlighting the process involved in changing the law**

Acknowledgement

Special thanks are due to Melanie Roberts for her help with the information on Scots law.

References

1. Salmond Sir John. Cited in Martin J. GCSE law. London: Hodder and Stoughton; 1995.
2. Labour Party Manifesto 1997. Online. Available: http://www.labour-party.org.uk/manifestos/1997/1997-labour-manifesto.shtml 12 May 2005.
3. Hunting Act 2004. London: HMSO.
4. Scotland Act 1998. London: HMSO.
5. Protection of Wild Mammals (Scotland) Act 2002. London: HMSO.
6. Judgment of Sheriff T.A.K. Drummond QC in the cause PF Jedburgh v Trevor Adams. Online. Available: http://www.scotcourts.gov.uk/opinions/adams.html. 23 Jun 2005.
7. DEFRA News Release. Scottish hunter would not be acquitted in England or Wales: Alun Michael. 14 Dec 2004. Online. Available: http://www.defra.gov.uk/news/2004/041214a.htm. 23 Jun 2005.

4
Negligence and whistle-blowing
Elizabeth Earle

NEGLIGENCE

Veterinary nurses have a duty in law not to cause harm or loss to clients. Animals count as property and any harm to them must, for an action in the tort of negligence to be successful, result in loss to the owner. An example would be damage to a pedigree cat which prevented the owner from showing and/or breeding from it.

In order for negligence to be established, three questions must be addressed:

1. Is there a 'duty of care'?
2. Has there been a breach of that duty of care?
3. Has this resulted in damage which would have been reasonably foreseeable?

Is there a duty of care?

In the case of R v. Bateman[1] the judge set a precedent by stating that 'If a person holds himself out as possessing a special skill and knowledge and is consulted as possessing such by or on behalf of a patient, he then owes a duty to the patient to use due caution in undertaking the treatment.'

Practice staff have an accepted duty of care to clients and colleagues; the question is more likely to be whether there has been a breach of that duty and whether this caused harm.

Veterinary nurses owe a duty of care to clients of the practice, their colleagues and their employer, and certain other individuals. It is important to recognise that, whatever the moral obligation is felt to be, there is no legal duty of care owed to an animal patient. The duty of care concerning an animal is owed to its owner.

A problem may arise where someone acts as a 'Good Samaritan' in an incident outside the practice environment, (for example by administering first aid) but inadvertently causes further injury. There is no legal obligation to provide care and treatment for a stranger. An individual, even a doctor, may walk past an accident with legal impunity.

This may seem odd. However, the law must respect an individual's right to judge whether or not they are competent to deal with a situation and to 'opt out' if they decide that they are not.

In contrast, the RCVS does not allow a veterinary surgeon to 'opt out'. It expects a veterinary surgeon to provide emergency treatment including first aid and pain relief to all species.[2] However, veterinary nurses have the same opportunity to 'opt out' as other members of the public.

Has there been a breach of that duty of care?

Once it has been established that a duty of care is owed, the injured party must be able to prove that there has been a breach of that duty of care. In order to do this, they must be able to show that the care or service provided fell below a reasonable standard of practice. The courts will decide what is a reasonable standard of practice by determining what the 'ordinary skilled professional' would have done in the circumstances of the case. A person who claims to have a special skill is judged according to the standard of the reasonable person who has that skill or qualification. The case would be supported by documentary evidence of the standard of competence required for registration.

Box 4.1

A veterinary nurse would be judged against the Veterinary Nursing Occupational Standard and advice from expert witnesses qualified to comment on standards of veterinary nursing competence.

Box 4.2 Bolam v. Friern Hospital Management Committee (1957)

A psychiatric patient was admitted for electro convulsive therapy (ECT) for depression which involves placing electrodes around the skull and passing an electric current through the brain. If no muscle relaxant is given violent fitting can occur. The patient was restrained by two nurses but flew from the couch and sustained bilateral hip fractures. The patient alleged that the doctor was negligent for not giving muscle relaxant and not providing adequate restraint. The judge decided that he was not negligent as there was a responsible body of medical opinion which would have acted in the same way.

The legal precedent for this comes from a medical case, Bolam v. Friern Hospital Management Committee,[3] which forms the basis for the 'Bolam test' which essentially provides that individuals will not be liable in negligence if they have demonstrably followed 'accepted practice'. In other words, professionals are judged against the standards of others undertaking similar work.

The Bolam test is the starting point in judging all cases of professional negligence. However, since that case, several questions have arisen regarding what constitutes acceptable practice. The courts accept that there are different ways of doing things and judges will not choose between different established professional opinions regarding acceptable practice.[4]

The most important challenge to the Bolam test in recent years has been the case of Bolitho v. City and Hackney Health Authority.[5] In this House of Lords case it was held that 'the judge, before accept-ing a body of opinion as being responsible, reasonable or respectable, will need to be satisfied . . . that the experts have weighed up the risks and benefits and have reached a defensible conclusion'. In other words, since the Bolitho case the courts have been more willing to be critical of 'accepted practice' and professionals must, accordingly, be prepared to present evidence-based practice.

In the National Health Service, clinical governance (the quality assurance processes such as clinical audit, risk management, etc.) and the National Institute for Clinical Excellence (NICE) clinical guidelines[6] will inevitably be used to challenge the Bolam test. Similar initiatives, which are key to measuring and improving standards of clinical practice, are also becoming established in veterinary practice and will increasingly provide the benchmarks for accepted practice.

Inexperience

Clients cannot be expected to distinguish between qualified or unqualified staff for themselves. In Wilsher v. Essex AHA[7] (a case concerning the negligence of a junior doctor), the judge said that: 'the law requires the trainee or learner to be judged by the same standard as his more experienced colleagues. If it did not, inexperience would frequently be urged as a defence to and action for professional negligence'. An individual must take responsibility for their own actions. Before undertaking any procedure they must ensure they have had sufficient training and have the correct skills, competence and authority to carry out the task.

Has this resulted in damage which would have been reasonably foreseeable?

The consequences of a negligent act must be foreseeable by a reasonable person in the given circumstances. However, the courts must decide how likely it would be that an action might cause harm; an individual cannot be expected to guard against an infinitesmal chance that something might pose a risk. It is important to recognise that, provided there is a foreseeable risk of harm, it does not matter that all the consequences are unforeseeable. As illustrated by the following case:

Box 4.3 The case of Bradford v. Robinson Rentals[8]

In this case a van driver's employers required him to drive from Bedford to Exeter on an exceptionally cold day in winter. There was no heater in the van. As a result of the cold, he suffered frostbite, a very rare condition in southern England. His employers were held liable, no matter that frostbite is rare or that the driver may have been unusually susceptible to it.

Box 4.4 Mahon v. Osbourne[9]

Swabs were left inside a patient during an operation. The patient could not explain exactly what happened but the 'facts spoke for themselves'.

Res ipsa loquitur: The facts speak for themselves

This phrase is applied where negligence is evident purely from the injury suffered by the plaintiff.

In order for res ipsa loquitur to apply, three conditions must be satisfied:

1. The defendant must be in control of the thing which caused injury to the claimant.
2. The accident must be of such a nature that it would not have occurred but for negligence.
3. There must be no acceptable explanation for the incident.

Causation and compensation

A claimant must establish that the harm or loss they have suffered has been caused by the negligence of the defendant. In establishing causation, the courts must take care to establish that the injury is not the result of a pre-existing condition. Sometimes it can be extremely difficult to establish the exact cause of an injury.

Box 4.5

Example: A client trips over a loose floor covering in the practice and injures her back. However, she has a previous history of back problems. In this case, the court would need to decide what proportion of the damage was due to the fall and how much was pre-existing.

An award of damages is made with the intention of restoring the injured party to the state they were in prior to the negligent act. The courts will compensate for loss of earnings, medical expenses and loss of property and will also allow damages for loss of future earnings and pension (in serious/long-lasting injury), pain, suffering and loss of amenity (the reduced ability to lead a normal life).

If an animal has been damaged or lost due to negligence by a veterinary practice, the owner may sue for the reduction in value or the loss of the animal, and to recover veterinary fees. As most pets are of limited financial value, it is often not worthwhile for the clients of small animal practices to sue. The situation is markedly different in equine practice where patients, and their earning potential, may be worth many thousands of pounds.

WHISTLE-BLOWING

While veterinary nurses are not yet professionally bound by a code of conduct, most would nonetheless agree that they have an ethical duty to uphold standards of care for their patients and clients, and to protect colleagues from abuse at work. This may sometimes lead to conflicts between the obligations of nurses to their employers on the one hand and the need to address poor standards of care or practice on the other. Many nurses experience these conflicts and yet feel powerless to do anything about them. Addressing such problems within any workplace is difficult, however; as employees in a small workplace, the staff of a veterinary practice understandably feel very vulnerable to a breakdown in working relationships or to loss of employment.

This difficulty affects the majority of staff working within veterinary practice, veterinary surgeons as well as veterinary nurses, students and lay staff. However, professional staff have a duty to uphold ethical standards of practice. They should not be intimidated into colluding with unacceptable practices or deliberately concealing their own mistakes. Personal fears will often need to be acknowledged and thought through in the process of dealing with moral conflicts in practice. Help is available, in the form of representative organisations.

The whistle-blowing procedure

There are three stages to the whistle-blowing procedure:

1. Try to reach an internal solution.
   - Concerns about standards of care should first be reported to the employer wherever possible, even if it seems likely that no action can or will be taken. Such reporting should be well considered and prepared; preferably with the help of some written notes. Advice from a professional association should be sought beforehand.

When raising issues of concern, examples of the practice in question should be given, preferably with as much detail as possible regarding when this occurred, along with the reasons for concern. Workable suggestions for improvements and change should be offered wherever possible so that the discussion may be seen to be constructive. If issues are raised verbally, it is wise to keep a written note of the date, issues discussed and the outcome for future reference.

2. Contacting the professional association.
   - Sometimes, despite discussing concerns with an employer, an employee may feel that no

progress has been made to address the issues raised. In this situation the next stage is to contact the professional regulatory body. Most professional bodies issue their members with advice in the form of a whistle-blowing procedure.

3. Going public.
   - If the situation remains unresolved, and is serious enough, an employee may consider disclosing their concerns publicly. One of the first, and widely publicised, incidents of whistle-blowing concerned Graham Pink, a charge nurse working on night duty in the NHS.[10]

The Pink case illustrates three essential elements of whistle-blowing:

1. The perception by someone within an organisation that something is amiss.
2. The communication of those concerns to outside parties.

Box 4.7

Currently the 'Guide to Professional Conduct for Veterinary Nurses' does not provide a protocol for whistle blowing. In view of this any veterinary nurse wishing to discuss a problem should contact the RCVS professional conduct department for advice. It is anticipated that a whistle-blowing procedure will be incorporated in future versions of the Guide to Professional Conduct.

Box 4.8

Graham Pink expressed concerns about low staffing levels and unacceptable standards of care to his employer, and subsequently at every management level including the Department of Health. No action was taken and, in desperation, he wrote to the local paper and made the matter public. He was sacked by his employers on the grounds that he had breached patient confidentiality, but later reinstated by an employment tribunal.

Box 4.6

The British Veterinary Nursing Association provides its members with a free helpline to advise on industrial relations

3. The perception by those in authority within the organisation that such a communication ought not to have been made.

The public disclosure of concerns about standards of care is an extreme step to take and the consequences for both the profession concerned and an employee may be far-reaching. Such a move may adversely affect public confidence in a profession or service. It is also likely to alienate an employee within the workplace and the employer could try to initiate disciplinary action. It is therefore essential to consider the justifiability of 'going public'. Whistle-blowing should only be considered when:

- It will lead to a review of procedures and policies.
- It serves some purpose in correcting or preventing poor practice.
- It will be done in a responsible manner.
- All other internal channels of complaint and redress have been exhausted.

Making an unauthorised public disclosure should always be the action of last resort when trying to address a major problem within veterinary practice. The Public Interest Disclosure Act 1998[11] provides protection from victimisation for employees who disclose concerns about breaches of law, e.g. dangers to health and safety or the environment.

References

1. R v. Bateman {1925} 94 LJKB 791.
2. RCVS Guide to professional conduct. London: RCVS; 2004.
3. Bolam v. Friern Hospital Management Committee {1957} 2 All ER 118.
4. Maynard v. West Midlands RHA {1985} 1 All ER 635.
5. Bolitho v. City and Hackney Health Authority {1997} [1998] Lloyd's Rep Med 26; [1998] AC 232.
6. National Institute for Clinical Excellence: Clinical guidance. Online. Available: http://www.nice.org.uk 19 May 2005.
7. Wilsher v. Essex AHA {1987} 2 WLR 425.
8. Bradford v. Robinson Rentals {1967}1 WLR 337.
9. Mahon v. Osbourne {1939}2 KB 141.
10. McHale J, Tingle J. Law and nursing. 2nd edn. Edinburgh: Butterworth Heinemann; 2003:150–151.
11. The Public Interest Disclosure Act 1998. London: HMSO.

Further reading

Dimond B. Legal aspects of nursing. 4th edn. London: Prentice Hall; 2004.

5
Regulation and representation
Sally Bowden and Sophie Pullen

Imagine a world where anybody can become a doctor or veterinary surgeon. They need not complete any training, or prove in any way that they are competent to practise. They can use whichever method of treatment they wish and charge any amount they choose for their services. If they do something wrong, there is no one the patient or owner can turn to for advice or redress and there is no method of preventing that person from continuing to practise. This is a world without regulation and in the early 1800s, this was reality!

The drive to regulate these professions initially came from those who had undergone some training, felt that they were practising competently, and wished to differentiate themselves from those who did not. This action was not entirely selfless as it also allowed an element of price-fixing and control over territory; the use of title and the right to practise was legally reserved for members of that profession – the 'professionals'.

This chapter explores the meaning, structure and role of regulation in today's world and provides a valuable insight for veterinary nurses, for whom regulation is looming.

It is also important to differentiate between the roles of a regulatory and representative body. This chapter clarifies these differences and highlights the importance of representation and the key roles of representative bodies.

WHAT IS REGULATION?

Today, the term 'professional' has come to mean many different things. For example, a 'professional footballer' is one who is paid to play football. The term, 'behaving in a professional manner' can be applied to anybody who demonstrates a certain standard of etiquette in the course of their work. It is important to acknowledge that being professional is not the same as being a member of a profession.

The public expects members of a profession to be knowledgeable and skilled in their role, to be motivated by a desire to help others and demonstrate a certain standard of behaviour. But what exactly is a profession?

The term 'profession' is not easily defined, although there is general agreement over the central features. Killeen[1] states that a profession is characterised by, 'prolonged education that takes place in a college or university and results in the acquisition of a body of knowledge based on theory and research. Values, beliefs, and ethics relating to the profession are an integral part of the education'. Hern[2] concurs with this view and adds that a profession is, 'a deliberate career choice rather than just a job – suggesting long-term commitment' and also agrees with Burnard and Chapman,[3] who state that, 'the attitude of the professional toward the client is one of service on an individual basis, the clients needs being placed before the professional'.

Perhaps the two key distinguishing characteristics of a profession are those of autonomy and accountability. Killeen[1] defines professional autonomy as, 'independence or the freedom to act. It implies control over practice and is exemplified by the profession being invested with responsibilities...' and goes on to define accountability as, 'the state of being responsible and answerable for one's own behaviour'. But how does a member of a profession know what their responsibilities are and how to behave? They clearly need guidelines and a set of rules within which they can operate; this is the basis of regulation.

Ogus[4] suggested that the term regulation should be used to indicate any form of control over behaviour, whatever the origin. In the context of professions, regulation is about exerting control over who may practise that profession – it is about setting and maintaining the standard at which one should work.

Regulation of a profession may be statutory (i.e. required by law) or voluntary. For example, there is a statutory requirement for veterinary surgeons to be registered with, and therefore regulated by, The Royal College of Veterinary Surgeons. This requirement is written into the Veterinary Surgeons Act 1966. The Association of Pet Behaviour Counsellors operates a 'Code of Practice' by which its members are bound, but it is perfectly legal to practice as a pet behaviour therapist without being a member. (Fig. 5.1)

WHY IS IT REQUIRED?

Historically, the aim of regulation may have been chiefly self-serving, but in the modern world the primary purpose of regulation must be to protect those who use the service offered. According to

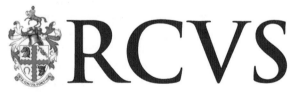

Royal College of Veterinary Surgeons

Figure 5.1 A register, whether it is statutory or voluntary, is different to the 'List of veterinary nurses' referred to in Schedule 3 of the Veterinary Surgeons Act 1966, held by the Royal College of Veterinary Surgeons. Currently, veterinary nurses pay an annual retention fee in order to maintain their listed status, thus allowing them to perform procedures described in the Act. Although nurses must satisfy certain criteria to enter the List, they are not beholden to any code of conduct or at risk of disciplinary proceedings.

Allsop and Mulcahy,[5] who examine the justification for regulation of the medical profession:

> Patient choice and information for patients as consumers have become more important. At the same time, the intimacy of the doctor–patient relationship, the potential for exploitation and the serious consequences of medical mistakes have all been given as justifications for regulation from a consumer perspective.

There have also been several high profile cases in the medical field, which have brought this issue to the fore. For example, following the inquiry into the deaths of patients at the hands of GP Dr Harold Shipman, Dame Janet Smith[6] commented on the General Medical Council (GMC), the regulatory body for doctors. She stated that, 'In the past, the GMC has been accountable to the public only in very general terms.' She suggested that some members of the GMC have favoured the interests of doctors over those of patients when specific issues arise. Dame Janet went on to say, 'To do their work properly as members of a regulatory body, they have to put the public interest first.'

With regard to veterinary nursing, the lack of a regulatory framework means that the consumer is not protected from poor veterinary nursing practice. There is no obligation for veterinary nurses to be Listed, unless they are performing procedures described in Schedule 3 of the Veterinary Surgeons Act. Even if a veterinary nurse is Listed, 'there is no legal way of ensuring that incompetent, criminal, or individuals otherwise unfit to practice, are removed from the List of veterinary nurses, or that nurses maintain their competence to practise'.[7] As veterinary nurses are not accountable for their conduct, they may be less likely to consider the consequences of their actions.

Statutory regulation means that members of that profession cannot practise unless they are registered with their professional body and abide by its code of conduct. The consumer can have confidence that the professional would not be offering their services unless this was the case. Voluntary regulation provides consumers with a choice – they could use the services of a non-registered person, or they could select a registered person where at least they have a measure of quality assurance. Of

Box 5.1

A dog is admitted to a veterinary hospital with a spinal injury resulting in quadriplegia and incontinence. It is not placed on the correct bedding and receives inadequate nursing care for several days. As a result, the dog develops decubitus ulcers and severe urine scalding.

Although this is clearly a nursing issue, according to current legislation the veterinary surgeon is responsible for the nurse's actions and omissions. If the client made a complaint to the RCVS, the veterinary surgeon and not the veterinary nurse involved would be held to account.

There is currently no mechanism by which the veterinary nurse could be held professionally accountable for their actions and omissions and notwithstanding any action taken by the employer, they could continue to practise veterinary nursing without addressing the situation surrounding the case.

course, the pitfall of a voluntary scheme is that consumers must be aware of its existence and understand its benefits.

Aside from protection of the consumer, there may be other reasons why the prospect of regulation is attractive to veterinary nurses. One such reason may be to enhance the status of the VN. The overwhelmingly positive response to the consultation paper regarding regulation published by the RCVS in 2003 may be as a result of this perception. Many veterinary nurses also aired their views when responding to the Veterinary Nursing Manpower Survey.[8] One respondent remarked:

> I feel very strongly that in order for veterinary nurses to acquire the recognition we want, and to be viewed as a profession, we need to accept that accountability and regulation is part and parcel of that.

Another reason for veterinary nurses to regard regulation as a positive move is its potential use as a lever for the development of a knowledge base. Regulatory bodies require the ongoing professional development of their members in order to protect the consumer. When discussing human nurses, Cormack[9] states:

A nurse who is oblivious to the latest available knowledge relevant to his or her area of practice, and uses redundant methods, cannot expect public trust and confidence and such a nurse will not enhance the good standing and reputation of the profession. The interests of society will not be served and interests of individual patients and clients will not be safeguarded.

While veterinary surgeons continue to be accountable for the actions of veterinary nurses, the development of veterinary nursing may be impeded as there is no incentive to develop a knowledge base.

THE STRUCTURE OF A REGULATORY BODY

In this country, professions are historically self-regulating, i.e. the rules are set, agreed and policed by members of the profession being regulated. This remains the case and is in contrast to the situation in many other countries, where state regulation, that is, regulatory systems run by government departments, is more common. However, some industries in the UK are regulated directly by agencies specially set up by government, for example Oftel, which regulates the telecommunications industry.

The remainder of this section essentially deals with self-regulation, as this is more pertinent to veterinary nursing. There are advantages and disadvantages to self-regulation over government intervention. Table 5.1 describes some of these.

Professions regulated by statute have a regulatory framework embedded in law. Legislation is not required for those who wish to set up a system of voluntary regulation. Until the Veterinary Surgeons Act 1966 is reformed or replaced, any regulatory scheme set up for veterinary nurses can only be voluntary.

Regardless of the nature of the profession and the form of regulation, regulatory bodies should take into account the key principles associated with professional regulation when considering their constitution. These were described by The Better Regulation Task Force,[10] an independent advisory body, which was established in 1997, and are outlined below.

Table 5.1 The advantages and disadvantages of self-regulation over government intervention

Advantages
Rules are developed by those involved in the profession and reflect the issues and needs of the sector.
Can generate a sense of ownership amongst the profession – more likely to secure a high level of compliance.
Easy to adapt and update to reflect changing circumstances and developments.
Self-regulation can provide a quicker and cheaper means of redress for the consumer.
It may be disproportionately expensive or difficult for government to acquire the specialist knowledge necessary to regulate effectively.
It can harness a close relationship between the profession and their clients.
Disadvantages
There is a danger of self-interest being put ahead of the public interest.
The organisation involved in enforcement may not be open and transparent about their processes and outcomes.
There may be a lack of public confidence in the ability of or the incentives for a self-regulatory body to provide effective consumer protection, and to impose appropriate sanctions when rules are broken.
Consumers may not be aware of who or what is regulated.

Box 5.2 The five key principles of good regulation

Proportionality – regulators should only intervene when necessary. Remedies should be appropriate to the risk posed, and costs identified and minimised. For example, enforcers should consider an educational, rather than punitive approach where possible.

Accountability – regulators must be able to justify decisions, and be subject to public scrutiny. For example, regulators and enforcers should establish clear standards and criteria against which they can be judged. Also, there should be well publicised, accessible, fair and effective complaints and appeals procedures.

Consistency – government rules and standards must be joined up and implemented fairly. For example, regulation should be predictable in order to give stability and certainty to those being regulated.

Transparency – regulators should be open, and keep regulation simple and user-friendly. For example, those being regulated should be made aware of their obligations, with law and best practice clearly distinguished. The consequences of non-compliance should be made clear.

Targeting – regulation should be focused on the problem, and minimise side-effects. For example, regulations should be systematically reviewed to test whether they are still necessary and effective. If not, they should be modified or eliminated.

All regulatory bodies, therefore, have the same basic 'ingredients' although their actual structures may differ. Generally, they consist of a central group of people – usually known as a 'council' or 'board' – which assumes overall responsibility for making decisions regarding matters of policy including the rules of regulation. People serving on a council are normally a mix of those elected by members of the profession, and those nominated by outside organisations. Nominated council members may or may not have voting rights. Some bodies have two groups of people, e.g. a council

---

Box 5.3   RCVS Veterinary Nurses Council

This Council evolved from the RCVS Veterinary Nursing Committee and was set up with the purpose of preparing for and undertaking voluntary regulation of veterinary nurses. In due course, it is anticipated that this body will also undertake the statutory regulation of veterinary nurses following legislative change.

At the current time the Veterinary Nurses Council is, strictly speaking, still a committee of the RCVS Council and has no regulatory powers. All decisions are subject to the approval of the RCVS Council.

The current structure of Veterinary Nurses Council is described below.

8 elected veterinary nurses
8 veterinary surgeons (members and non-
   members of the RCVS Council)
2 lay members
Chairman of the National Training Organisation
   for Professions Allied to Veterinary Science
1 representative from BVNA (non-voting)
1 representative from BSAVA (non-voting)

---

and a board, the terms of reference for each being defined in the constitution of the body involved.

The actual composition of a council varies between individual regulatory bodies. The number of people serving on these may be determined by statute, for example the Veterinary Surgeons Act 1966, which describes the number and types of people required to form the Royal College of Veterinary Surgeons Council (Table 5.2). Some regulatory bodies are responsible for more than one profession. An example of this is the Health Professions Council, which regulates thirteen different professions (Table 5.2).

One feature common to all councils is the inclusion of lay representation. A lay member is essentially one who is independent from the profession, and who should have no vested interest in agreeing or disagreeing with the views of the other members of that council. They are present to provide a more balanced discussion of any issues and offer an 'out-siders' viewpoint. Lay members may be retired professionals, academics associated with the profession, representatives of other industries or they may be consumers – members of the public who have no specialist knowledge of the profession at all. Some bodies specify which 'type' of lay member they should have on their council – others do not specify this.

The amount of lay representation on councils is a contentious issue. The Better Regulation Task Force[10] states that lay representation on decision-making bodies is needed, 'to ensure that a balance is struck between bringing expertise to bear and the need to challenge professional complacency'. Over recent years, there has been a trend towards increasing the percentage of lay representation. The National Consumer Council[11] recommend they should be in the majority – 'if possible, up to 75 percent'. However, recently regulated professions have favoured a lay representation of around 50%. The NCC go on to say that, 'Schemes should avoid the temptation to "window-dress" with one or two consumer representatives without wide-ranging expertise or access to research and other resources' and 'where there is no lay majority, then some regular outside scrutiny may be necessary to maintain consumer confidence'. It is sometimes necessary for lay people to attend specialist courses in order that they can fully understand the issues under debate.

Regulatory bodies all function using a series of committees, which undertake much of the debating, formulating and instigating of policies deemed necessary by the council. It is standard practice for the committees to make recommendations to the council, which may then approve or not approve these recommendations. Committees may be statutory, i.e. described within the legislation relating to that profession, or they may be non-statutory, i.e. deemed necessary by the regulatory body but not required by law. Some committees are long-standing and others may be convened and disbanded as the need arises. Committees usually comprise a number of council members, selected professionals who may be specialists in the subject area and a number of other interested parties. They may also include lay members.

Table 5.2 shows the committees of various councils.

Table 5.2 Examples of regulatory frameworks for various professional bodies

Professional body	Profession/s regulated	Number serving on council	Statutory committees	Non-statutory committees
Royal College of Veterinary Surgeons	Veterinary surgeons	40 members 24 veterinary surgeons 4 members elected by the Privy Council (The Chief Veterinary Officer plus 3 lay members) 2 representatives from each veterinary school	Preliminary Investigation Committee Disciplinary Committee Registration Appeals Committee	Advisory Committee Education Committee Examination Appeals Committee External Affairs Committee Finance and General Purposes Committee Nominations Committee Specialisation and Further Education Committee VN Council
Farriers Registration Council	Farriers	16 members 3 persons appointed by The Worshipful Company of Farriers 2 self-employed farriers 2 employed farriers 2 persons from National Master Farrier Blacksmith and Agricultural Engineering Association 2 persons appointed by the RCVS 1 lay representative appointed by each of the following*: Jockey Club RSPCA British Equestrian Federation Council for Small Industries in Rural Areas Council for Small Industries in Rural Areas of Scotland *cannot be a Registered Farrier or Veterinary Surgeon	Investigating Committee Disciplinary Committee	Finance Committee Registration Committee Joint Farriery Training Committee

Table 5.2 Examples of regulatory frameworks for various professional bodies – cont'd

Professional body	Profession/s regulated	Number serving on council	Statutory committees	Non-statutory committees
The Health Professions Council	Arts therapists Biomedical scientists Chiropodists/ podiatrists Clinical scientists Dieticians Occupational therapists Operating department practitioners Orthoptists Paramedics Physiotherapists Prosthetists/orthotists Radiographers Speech and language therapists	26 members 1 representative from each profession 13 lay member	Investigating Committee Conduct and Competence Committee Health Committee Education and Training Committee	Finance and Resources Committee Communications Commitee Registration Committee
The Nursing and Midwifery Council	Nurses Midwives	23 members 12 professionals 11 lay members	Health Committee Preliminary Proceedings Committee Professional Conduct Committee Midwifery Committee	Standards Committee Communications Committee Audit Committee Recruitment and Appointments Committee Finance and Business Planning Committee Human Resources Committee

Members of councils or committees are expected to comply with the seven Principles of Public Life as described by the Nolan Committee's Report into Standards in Public Life[12] (Table 5.3).

THE ROLE OF A REGULATORY BODY

The function of any regulatory body remains essentially the same – to protect the consumer by setting and maintaining the standards for registered professionals. Within this remit, it is possible to identify key functions:

- Holding and maintaining a register.
- Setting standards for education, practice and conduct.
- Maintaining standards, i.e. considering allegations of misconduct or unfitness to practice due to ill health, monitoring CPD and returning to practice.
- Providing advice for professionals and consumers.

Holding and maintaining a register

This role falls to the registrar, a person usually appointed by the council of the regulatory body.

Table 5.3 The seven principles of public life

Selflessness	Holders of public office should take decisions solely in terms of the public interest. They should not do so in order to gain financial or other material benefits for themselves, their family, or their friends.
Integrity	Holders of public office should not place themselves under any financial or other obligations to outside individual organisations that might influence them in the performance of their official duties.
Objectivity	In carrying out public business, including making public appointments, awarding contracts, or recommending individuals for rewards and benefits, holders of public office should make choices on merit.
Accountability	Holders of public office are accountable for their decisions and actions to the public and must submit themselves to whatever scrutiny is appropriate to their office.
Openness	Holders of public office should be as open as possible about all the decisions and actions that they take. They should give reasons for their decisions and restrict information only when the wider public interest demands.
Honesty	Holders of public office have a duty to declare any private interests relating to their public duties and to take steps to resolve any conflicts arising in a way that protects the public interest.
Leadership	Holders of public office should promote and support these principles by leadership and example.

The council prescribes the fees for retention on, and restoration to, the register, and informs the registrar who is eligible for entry. They may also specify which additional qualifications can be cited in the register.

The registrar is responsible for ensuring that the register is up to date and accurate, printed and published in accordance with the wishes of the council. The frequency of publication may be described in statute. Most professional bodies have internet sites, where it is possible for the public to access their register electronically.

Setting standards

Education
The council of a professional body, usually through an education committee, establishes the minimum requirements for entry onto their register. This always includes a requirement for registrants to hold a formal qualification, for example, a degree. It may also necessitate the undertaking of a specified amount or type of experience in the workplace, which may be necessary before or after

Box 5.4

For veterinary nurses, the minimum requirements for entry onto the List are laid out in the National Occupational Standards. These are written following consultation with the veterinary and veterinary nursing industries and are designed to reflect the current needs of employers and the consumer.

Currently, the only qualifications that are recognised by the RCVS are the National Vocational Qualifications Levels 2 and 3 in Veterinary Nursing, for which the RCVS is the only awarding body. These are assessed against the agreed National Occupational Standards. However, pilot schemes are running to investigate the possibility that some higher education programmes may also meet the Standards. Should these be successful, this would be a second route of entry onto the List. (Table 5.4)

registration. Most registers have a variety of categories, for example, provisional, overseas or limited registrations to cater for those who may not be eligible to practise without restriction.

Table 5.4 Entry requirements of various professional bodies

Profession	Academic requirements	Pre-registration work experience	Post-registration work experience
Nurses	Recognised qualification	Certain time requirements written into academic modules	None
Doctors	Recognised degree	Certain time requirements written into academic modules	1 year whilst provisionally registered
Veterinary surgeons	Degree recognised by the RCVS	Degree programmes have a requirement for completion of work experience (Extra Mural Studies – EMS)	None (there is currently a move to change this)
Veterinary Nurses (entry onto RCVS List)	Completion of NVQ levels 2 and 3 in Veterinary Nursing	Completion of 94 full-time weeks (or equivalent) working as student veterinary nurse in an approved Training Practice	None

Practice and conduct

It has been established that in order for professionals to know what their responsibilities are and how to behave, they need a set of rules and guidelines within which they can operate. These rules are laid out in professional codes. There are two sorts of code, a 'code of ethics' and a 'code of professional conduct'.

Rumbold[13] states, 'A code of ethics is a statement of belief. It is a statement about what the profession believes itself and its purpose to be, and, therefore, embodies a statement of belief about human nature.' Not all professional bodies publish a code of ethics. Some bodies may incorporate ethical beliefs within a code of conduct.

Rumbold goes on to say, 'A code of conduct is a framework for behaviour. It is a statement about how the profession considers its members should behave toward clients, society as a whole and each other.' Burnard and Chapman[14] concur with this view, saying that a code of conduct is 'a code of guidance regarding appropriate conduct for a specific group of people carrying out specific actions'.

All professions have either a code of conduct or a guide to conduct. Breach of a code of conduct will almost invariably lead to disciplinary action, whereas breach of a guide to conduct, although it may be used as evidence in any disciplinary pro-

Box 5.5

Veterinary nurses currently do have a 'Guide to Professional Conduct' (Appendix 1). However, this is very brief and unfortunately, does not provide particularly clear guidance. In places, it is also contradictory to the guidance given in the RCVS Guide to Professional Conduct for veterinary surgeons. If a veterinary nurse was accused of breaching this Guide, there is little the RCVS can do in the way of investigation or disciplinary action. This situation would change if veterinary nurses were regulated on a voluntary or statutory basis.

cedure does not automatically result in disciplinary action.

They usually follow a similar format, being comprised of a set of key statements, which are then expanded upon. An example of the standard format for codes of conduct is given in the Table 5.5.

According to the NMC,[15] the purpose of a code of conduct is to:

- Inform the professions of the standard of professional conduct required of them in the exercise of their professional accountability.

Table 5.5 Extract from The Nursing and Midwifery Council (NMC): Code of Professional Conduct[15]

Key statement	4. As a registered nurse, midwife or health visitor, you must co-operate with others in the team.
Expansion of key statement	4.1 The team includes the patient or client, the patient's or client's family, informal carers and health and social care professionals in the National Health Service, independent and voluntary sectors.
	4.2 You are expected to work co-operatively within teams and to respect the skills, expertise and contributions of your colleagues. You must treat them fairly and without discrimination.
	4.3 You must communicate effectively and share your knowledge, skill and expertise with other members of the team as required for the benefit of patients and clients.
Further guidance	Available from the Nursing and Midwifery Council.

- Inform the public, other professions and employers of the standard of professional conduct that they can expect of a registered practitioner.

However, according to Rumbold,[16] 'Professional codes cannot and do not provide answers to every situation . . . The purpose of professional codes is to enable members of a profession to exercise accountability and responsibility, and not to dictate actions.'

Maintaining standards

Continuing professional development (CPD)
It is important to realise that, 'clinical knowledge does not stand still'.[3] Professional bodies usually require members of their profession to undertake CPD in order that they '. . . maintain, enhance and broaden their competence to practise. It is a systemic and cyclical process that is undertaken throughout an individual's career to develop and enhance performance at work'.[17] Similarly, it is generally accepted that those returning to practice following a significant break will need to update their practical skills and theoretical knowledge.

There are several different ways by which CPD can be achieved and recorded. Each regulatory body decides on acceptable methods. Human nurses, for example, must undertake PREP (Post Registration Education and Practice), amounting to 35 hours over a three-year period. Appropriate CPD activities include:

- Attendance at conferences/congresses.
- Additional qualifications – diplomas, degrees, etc.
- Attendance on courses.
- Personal study and reflection.
- Reading.
- Mentoring – a process using an experienced nurse who can offer help and support in a clinical setting.

Nurses must record their CPD using a template provided by the Nursing and Midwifery Council (NMC). This is subject to audit when they re-register.

In contrast, there is no mandatory CPD requirement for veterinary surgeons. However, the RCVS[18] recognises that, 'National and international demand and need for the development and maintenance of advanced clinical skills necessitate lifelong learning on behalf of all members of the profession.'

They recommend an average of 35 hours per annum over a three year period, 10 of which can be, 'informal distance learning and home study'. In 1997, a scheme of self-recording using a record card was introduced. This situation is likely to change and in all probability, mandatory CPD will be introduced when legislation is reviewed.

Box 5.6

Although there is currently no requirement for veterinary nurses to undertake CPD, the RCVS[19] acknowledges that, 'continuing professional development is key to ensuring that members of a profession retain the knowledge and skills expected of them by the public'. In anticipation of a scheme of voluntary regulation, the Veterinary Nurses Council debated a proposal for a CPD framework in February 2005.[19]

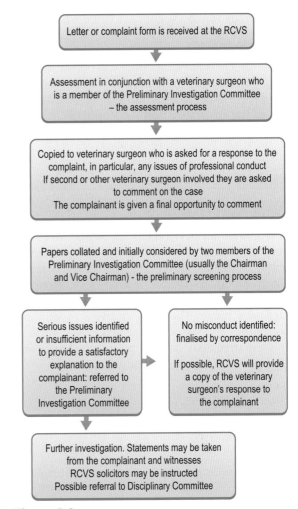

Figure 5.2

Disciplinary systems

All regulatory bodies have a system by which allegations against members of its profession can be investigated and, if necessary, action can be taken. Such action should have the primary aim of protecting the public from an incompetent or negligent practitioner, rather than 'punishing' the professional.

For this reason, modern thinking tends to favour measures such as recommending retraining and supervised practice rather than fining the professional involved. The removal of the professional's name from the register temporarily or permanently is still carried out when it is felt that the consumer is at significant risk.

If a professional is found to be in breach of their code of conduct, the focus should be on the circumstances surrounding the breach and the aim should be to prevent a reoccurrence. Many professional bodies incorporate a 'whistle-blowing' policy into their codes of conduct. This is in sharp contrast to the traditional view of reporting the mistakes and deficiencies in the work of fellow professionals. Dame Janet Smith comments on this in her report following the inquiry into the deaths of patients at the hands of GP Dr Harold Shipman[6] stating:

> It has always been possible for a doctor who was concerned about the treatment given to a patient by another doctor to report his/her concerns about that treatment to an appropriate authority. However, many doctors were not prepared to do that; they had been 'brought up' to regard it as improper to criticise or depreciate the conduct of a fellow professional. The culture was that it was 'not done'.

There is also more awareness of the impact health issues may have on a professional's ability to practise. Many regulatory bodies have a separate health committee, which deals with issues such as alcoholism and drug addiction amongst its members and may recommend treatment or counselling following a breach of the code of conduct.

Most professional bodies have similar components in their disciplinary systems, although the number and types of people sitting on the different committees varies considerably. Figure 5.2 depicts the RCVS complaints procedure for veterinary surgeons. Professional bodies must take into account The Human Rights Act 1998, which guarantees, 'the right to a fair and public hearing before an independent tribunal within a reasonable time whenever a person's civil rights and obligations are being determined'. This means that the disciplinary process must, to a certain extent, be independent of the council setting the standards.

REPRESENTATION

What is representation?

To 'represent' means to act as a substitute or proxy. A representative is an authorised delegate, agent, person or thing that represents another. A representative body is therefore a body or group of people who act as a voice for, in this instance, the veterinary nurse. The body is there to promote the feelings and wishes of the veterinary nurse. A representative body has the 'power' to change and influence whereas one individual may not.

The role of a representative body

The role of a representative body is very different to that of a regulatory body. Table 5.6 compares the role of each.

Some representative bodies are also unions, although essentially they have similar roles. The Royal College of Nursing (RCN) is the leading professional union for human nurses in the United Kingdom, describing itself as 'the voice of nursing'. Their mission statement is, 'The RCN represents nurses and nursing, promotes excellence in practice and shapes health policies.'[20] The British Veterinary Association which is the representative body for veterinary surgeons, is not a union, and refers to itself as 'the voice of the British veterinary profession'.[21]

Table 5.7 describes some of the differences between union and non-union representative bodies.

In the United Kingdom, The British Veterinary Nursing Association (BVNA) is the representative body for veterinary nurses. (Fig. 5.3)

Table 5.6   A table to compare the role of a regulatory body and a representative body

	Regulatory body	Representative body
How they are established	At government request, possibly led by a profession.	At the request of a profession/group of professional people.
Reason for being	To protect the consumer by setting and maintaining the standards for registered professionals.	To act as a voice for a profession, or for specified areas of a profession.
Setting standards		
Education	Responsible for setting the standards required for registration.	May offer careers advice and educational support.
Code of conduct	Formulates and enforces codes of practice.	Provides advice to professionals in the form of 'help lines' and associated literature.
Maintaining standards		
CPD	Sets and upholds the requirements for CPD in order to maintain registration.	Links CPD courses to the needs and requests of the profession.
Disciplinary procedure	Instigates and implements disciplinary process.	Represents professionals and provides legal advice. Some provide indemnity insurance.

Table 5.7 The differences between union and non-union representative bodies

Issue	Union	Non union
Law	Employment law states that only a trade union representative or a fellow employee can accompany a defendant at an employment tribunal.	A representative body can provide a service to a defendant by instructing them on the procedure to be undertaken, completing relevant documentation and putting forward a case, but would not be able to sit with them during the tribunal.
Political	Initially set up by members of the Labour party. The 'power' of a union is often dependant on the views of the government at a given time.	No political persuasion.
Cost	Joining a union often incurs additional costs.	Often cheaper than joining a union.
Type	A union may represent a variety of professions. Only industries with large numbers of workers will have their own union.	Specific to the profession it is serving. Often serve smaller industries/professions.

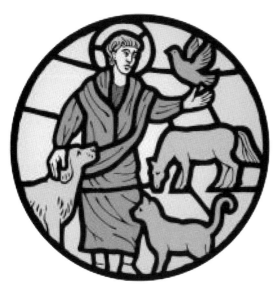

Figure 5.3 The image of St Francis appears on the BVNA logo and membership badge, an image that is also found on the Veterinary Nursing Badge produced by the RCVS.

THE HISTORY OF THE BVNA

Soon after the first veterinary nurses qualified (originally known as 'RANAs' – Registered Animal Nursing Auxiliaries (see Chapter 1), it was realised that there needed to be a method of liaison with the veterinary profession and a way of communicating with other RANAs and students. Initially, a small group of people got together and produced a 'newsletter', described by Mrs Townson, the first chairman of the BVNA, as a 'primitive affair'.[22] The newsletter was expensive to produce and as there were no funds available. Its production relied on the generosity of employers and supporters at the time.

It was then that the late Mr John Hodgman, MRCVS, suggested that an association should be formed with an elected council and a constitution. Mrs Townson admitted that none of the RANAs had 'any idea of committee procedure or how to set about forming an association'[22] and so elicited the help of Mr Alastair Porter, the Registrar of the RCVS at that time.

The BVNA was formed in 1965 but due to the fact that the title 'nurse' was protected by law under the Nurses, Midwives and Health Visitors Act (1979) and the title 'veterinary' was equally protected by charter,[22] it shortly changed its name to The British Animal Nursing Auxiliary Association (BANAA) and it was not until 1985 that the name returned to the original of BVNA.

The first meeting was attended by two veterinary surgeons and twenty-eight RANAs. Meetings were initially held in members' homes, waiting rooms, etc. before the British Veterinary Association offered the BVNA the use of one of its boardrooms at its headquarters in London for a Saturday morning meeting. By 1988 membership numbers had grown sufficiently to allow the association to rent its own premises.[23] The first headquarters of the BVNA was officially opened on Monday 15 August of that year.

The work of the BVNA is funded by its members. The BVNA currently has 4300 members (November 2004) and nine membership categories. It is thanks to the many RANAs and veterinary nurses who give up their time voluntarily that the BVNA has grown so significantly and achieved so much since its formation.

The work of the BVNA

The mission statement of the BVNA states that the Association represents veterinary nurses, a statement that does not do the Association justice as it also represents practice support staff such as receptionists. The work that the BVNA does can be compared to that of the RCN. (Table 5.8)

Table 5.8 A table to compare the aims of The Royal College of Nursing with the services provided by The British Veterinary Nursing Association

A list of aims devised by the RCN in order to fulfil their mission statement	The Royal College of Nursing The RCN represents nurses and nursing, promotes excellence in practice and shapes health policies	The British Veterinary Nursing Association Representing Veterinary nursing
Represent	Represent the interests of nurses and nursing and be their voice locally, nationally and internationally.	• Produce the Veterinary Nursing Journal (VNJ), which is distributed to all members. • The BVNA has carried out and continues to carry out market research aimed at identifying the needs of its members, allowing it to represent the views of veterinary nurses and produce constructive feedback, answer questions, highlight the concerns of its members. • The BVNA has a system of local/area representatives whose role is to liaise with members locally and provide CPD courses at a local level. • Has links with the International Veterinary Nurses and Technicians Association (IVNTA) and attends international conferences.
Influence	Influence and lobby governments and others to develop and implement policy that improves the quality of patient care and builds on the importance of nurses, health care assistants and nursing students to health outcomes.	• Has a non-voting representative on the RCVS Veterinary Nurses Council. • Is often representing veterinary nursing at local and national events relating to the veterinary and animal care industries.

Table 5.8 A table to compare the aims of The Royal College of Nursing with the services provided by The British Veterinary Nursing Association – cont'd

A list of aims devised by the RCN in order to fulfil their mission statement	The Royal College of Nursing The RCN represents nurses and nursing, promotes excellence in practice and shapes health policies	The British Veterinary Nursing Association Representing Veterinary nursing
Support and protect	Support and protect the value of nurses and nursing in all their diversity. Support and protect their terms and conditions of employment in all employment sectors. Support and protect the interests of nurses professionally.	• Providing fact sheets and publications giving advice on areas such as employment law including working time regulations, contracts of employment, maternity leave and bullying. • Support in the form of a free industrial relations service for its members. • Support in the form of a free telephone legal help line, email help line for its members. • Professional indemnity insurance.
Develop	Develop and educate nurses professionally and academically, building their resource of professional expertise and leadership.	• Since 1973 the BVNA has hosted an annual congress providing not only CPD but a chance for members to meet with other members, pose questions in an open forum and honour those that have been awarded prizes. In 2004 approximately 1200 veterinary nurses attended the conference. • In 2000 the BVNA CPD portfolio was designed highlighting the profession's desire to make sure that nurses keep up to date with their training and strive to maintain high levels of competence. • The BVNA offer a number of specialised courses for example, pharmacy management for veterinary nurses and the veterinary nurse certificate in dentistry. • The BVNA developed and administer the Animal Nursing Assistant qualification and also developed the original Advanced Diploma in Veterinary Nursing. • An array of bursaries is available to a range of different categories of BVNA member.

Table 5.8 A table to compare the aims of The Royal College of Nursing with the services provided by The British Veterinary Nursing Association – cont'd

A list of aims devised by the RCN in order to fulfil their mission statement	The Royal College of Nursing The RCN represents nurses and nursing, promotes excellence in practice and shapes health policies	The British Veterinary Nursing Association Representing Veterinary nursing
	Develop the science and art of nursing and its professional practice.	• In 2003 the BVNA formed a committee to look into VN research and as a result the BVNA now offers a grant to assist veterinary nurses to perform research aimed at moving the profession forwards and highlighting the need for evidence-based practice.
Build	Build a sustainable, member led, organization with the capacity to deliver their mission effectively, efficiently and in accordance with their values. Build the systems, attitudes and resources to offer the best possible support and development to their staff.	• All members of BVNA Council are elected by BVNA members. • Strong volunteer support is provided by the BVNA Council and committee members.

The Veterinary Nursing Journal

In 1970, the precursor to the current veterinary nursing journal, the BANNA Newsletter, was circulated. In 1972, the first Veterinary Nursing Journal was produced and in 1991 the first colour journal was issued. The newsletters and journals provide a communication tool and highlight aspects of the work of the BVNA together with current, important and topical issues and educational articles. (Fig. 5.4)

THE IMPORTANCE OF REPRESENTATION FOLLOWING REGULATION

It is not a requirement for nurses to be members of a representative body, but the benefits of becoming a member are clear. When regulation is introduced, these benefits will become more apparent. It is envisaged that areas of support such as the industrial relations service will be utilised more by veterinary nurses who need advice but do not want to contact the regulatory body.

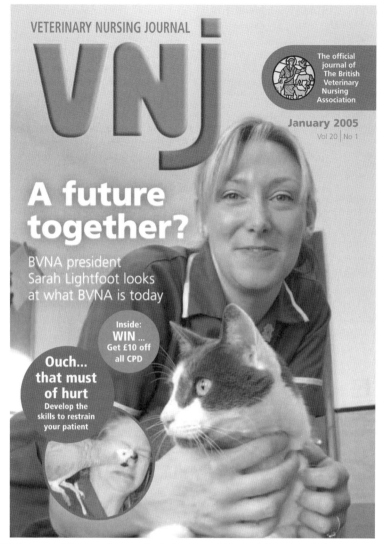

Figure 5.4 **The VNJ (copy of journal cover).** In January 2005 publication of the Veterinary Nursing Journal, 'VNJ' as it is now known, was taken over by the JCA Group and is now a monthly magazine (copyright applied for).

References

1. Killeen ML. Socialization to professional nursing. In: Creasia JL, Parker B, eds. Conceptual foundations: the bridge to professional nursing practice. 3rd edn. St Louis: Mosby; 2001:47–55.
2. Hern JC. Professional conduct and self regulation. In: Legood G, ed. Veterinary ethics: an introduction. London: Continuum; 2000: 64.
3. Burnard P, Chapman C. Professional and ethical issues in nursing. 3rd edn. Edinburgh: Bailliere Tindall; 2003:123.
4. Ogus A. Regulation: legal form and economic theory. Oxford: Clarendon Press; 1994.
5. Allsop J, Mulcahy L. Regulating medical work: formal and informal controls. Buckingham: Open University Press; 1996:12.
6. Smith J. The Shipman inquiry: independent public inquiry into the issues arising from the case of Harold Fredrick Shipman. Command

Paper CM 6394; 2004. Online. Available: http://www.the-shipman-inquiry.org.uk/5r_page.asp 17 Apr 2005.

7. Earle E. The case for regulation: developing veterinary nurse accountability. In: RCVS Veterinary Nursing News 1999; (2): November 4–5.

8. LANTRA, BVA, SPVS, BVNA, RCVS, BSAVA. Veterinary nursing manpower survey. Coventry: LANTRA; 2004.

9. Cormack D, ed. The Research process in nursing. 4th edn. Oxford: Blackwell Science; 2000:52.

10. Better Regulation Task Force: Principles of good regulation. 2003. Online: Available: http://www.brtf.gov.uk/docs/pdf/self regulation.pdf 4 May 2005.

11. The National Consumer Council: Three steps to credible self-regulation. 2003. Online: Available: http://www.ncc.org.uk 4 May 2005.

12. Nolan Committee. First report on standards in public life. London HMSO; 1995.

13. Rumbold G. Ethics in nursing and midwifery practice. London: Distance Learning Centre, South Bank Polytechnic; 1991.

14. Burnard P, Chapman C. Professional and ethical issues in nursing. Chichester: John Wiley; 1988.

15. The Nursing and Midwifery Council. Code of professional conduct. In Burnard P, Chapman C. Professional and ethical issues in nursing. 3rd edn. Edinburgh: Bailliere Tindall; 2003:123.

16. Rumbold G. Ethics in nursing practice. 3rd edn. Edinburgh: Bailliere Tindall; 2003:259.

17. Chartered Society of Physiotherapy. Core standards of physiotherapy practice: continuing professional development/lifelong learning. London: CSP; 2000.

18. RCVS Specialisation and Further Education Committee. Continuing professional development policy. London: RCVS; 2003.

19. RCVS Veterinary Nursing News 2005; 13: April.

20. Royal College of Nursing. Our mission. Online: Available http://www.rcn.org.uk/aboutus/mission.php 7 Jan 2005.

21. British Veterinary Association. About the BVA. Online. Available: http://www.bva.co.uk/about/about.html 8 Jan 2005.

22. Townson J. Cited in: Turner T. ed. Veterinary nursing: the first twenty five years. Harlow: British Veterinary Nursing Association; 1986:24.

23. Turner J. The evolution of veterinary nursing. The Veterinary Nursing Journal 1994; 9(4):107.

Further reading

The Human Rights Act 1998. London: HMSO.
Veterinary Surgeons Act 1966. London: HMSO.

6
The history of animal welfare
Pippa Swan

The legal and moral status of animals in society can only really be understood by looking at how the two have evolved. There are many anomalies and inconsistencies in the way that we currently regard animals, and these are explained, at least to a certain extent, by their historical context. By looking at where legislation governing the treatment of animals started from, we will be better equipped to apply our modern knowledge to the legal process. We also need to examine what we actually mean by the terms 'animal welfare', 'suffering' and 'cruelty' since they are referred to so widely, by those working with animals, and by those who express concern about their wellbeing.

WHAT IS WELFARE?

The word welfare is so commonly used when talking about how we do or should treat animals, that to many people its definition may seem obvious. Most of us are referring to an animal's quality of life, or a similar concept, when discussing welfare. In academic circles, however, a single definition of the term has yet to be agreed, and its use in law is relatively recent and still without a clear and precise meaning. Broadly speaking, definitions range from those with an emphasis on measurable physical and physiological factors, to those which focus more on feelings and psychological states. Parameters such as heart rate, growth rate, levels of blood cortisol and immune status can all be objectively monitored, and used to reach conclusions about how well an animal is doing in any particular situation. For example, welfare scientists, such as Broom and Johnson, are keen to

define welfare in terms of what can be measured and therefore clearly demonstrated.

> Welfare can be measured in a scientific way that is independent of moral considerations. Welfare measurements should be based on a knowledge of the biology of the species and, in particular, on what is known of the methods used by animals to try and cope with difficulties and signs that coping attempts are failing. The measurement and its interpretation should be objective. Once the welfare has been described, moral decisions can be taken.[1]

Others, however, approach welfare from a more feelings–based perspective; how animals actually feel about and perceive their situation. Dawkins, for example, stated, 'To be concerned about animal welfare is to be concerned with the subjective feelings of animals, particularly the unpleasant subjective feelings of suffering and pain.'[2] Duncan goes even further and asserts that, 'Neither health nor lack of stress nor fitness is necessary and/or sufficient to conclude that an animal has good welfare. Welfare is dependent on what animals feel'.[3]

Health is obviously key to both approaches of defining welfare since animals in poor health cannot be said to be 'coping' with life successfully, and are likely to 'feel' unwell or in pain as a result. In practical terms, however, neither model is mutually exclusive, and many methods of animal welfare assessment rely on both objective and subjective observations to varying degrees. Care must be taken, though, to recognise which types of measurement are being used to reach any conclusion regarding an animal's welfare. During an assessment, have established measures of health or physiological state been used (e.g. a diagnostic test showing an abnormality), or has an interpretation of an animal's behaviour, based on experience and informed opinion (e.g. shying away and crying out when a part of the body is touched), been used? Subjective statements about an animal's quality of life are valid when recognised criteria and evidence are used, but should be distinguished from those based on objective fact.

Death, euthanasia and killing are often emotive issues for those caring for animals and can confuse debates about animal welfare. The phrase 'death is not a welfare issue' is used by those keen to distinguish human and animal concerns, and usefully separates welfare from death. How an animal dies is obviously of great relevance to its welfare, but assuming a death to be painless and without unpleasant sensations then does it compromise welfare? In western cultures, most of us believe that killing to relieve suffering is a humane act, but what about killing where suffering is not present, to provide food or pleasure? How does that fit in with our feelings, often caring feelings, about animals? The killing of animals is justified using a variety of means: animals have no concept of death or the future; provided there is a good enough reason it's acceptable; some animals are bad or stupid, and so don't really matter. In fact, both as a society and as individuals, we tend to be inconsistent when it comes to animals and death. Instinctively, our reaction to the killing of a six month old, healthy dog, by an owner who has become bored by it, is likely to be very different from that to the killing of a six month old, healthy pig in a slaughter house to make bacon, an act which occurs on a massive scale every day. Our own feelings about the situation make little difference to the animal in question and these human concerns should be clearly distinguished from those of the animal.

WHAT IS SUFFERING?

Welfare can range from excellent to very poor. At some point indifferent or poor welfare may further deteriorate and cross an arbitrary line, which neither the legislators nor the courts have adequately defined, into the realms of suffering. Most of us would accept that animals, as indeed ourselves, do not spend their whole lives in a state of contentment and bliss. There will be short-term difficulties and discomforts, which are unpleasant, but would not be regarded as actual suffering. Indeed, the point at which suffering is reached might vary between individuals in very similar situations, and is likely to be affected by how an animal feels at the time. An injury sustained during an exciting or rewarding activity will produce different feelings from that sustained during a frightening or dreaded activity. Similarly, an animal who is in pain or feeling unwell, but is in a safe, warm and comfortable environment, will feel rather different from the animal with the same condition who is cold, frightened and away from familiar objects or companions. We might conclude that the animal in the first scenario has poor welfare, but that the animal in the second is suffering.

The examples above demonstrate a potential pitfall when assessing welfare and suffering in animals. It is easy to superimpose our own subjective feelings about an animal's situation onto any assessment. The animal described above in the warm and safe environment could be in the attentive care of a kind veterinary nurse, for example. It would be tempting, therefore, to assume that that animal *must* feel better, because our intentions regarding it are so well meant. In fact, it may still feel great pain and distress, in spite of, and sometimes because of (in the case of wild animals) our best efforts. Where animals are much loved by humans, it is particularly difficult to separate how an animal is doing and feeling from our own feelings and wishes. The old or terminally ill pet, which owners cannot bear to part with, is a common situation. So, too, is the elevation of certain types of animal to greater consideration and concern. Farmed animals, rats and other 'pests' generally do not fall into a category of animals about which we are sentimental, and so are treated very differently from those, like dogs and horses, which we regard as having a special status in society.

Broom and Johnson use a definition of suffering, which is that: 'suffering is an unpleasant subjective feeling which is prolonged or severe'.[1] But we are still left with the problem of what constitutes prolonged (hours, days, weeks?) and severe (pain which evokes a vocal response, isolation for a social animal?). The importance of our defining the word 'suffering' lies in its common use in the wording of legislation. Causing an animal to suffer unnecessarily constitutes a criminal offence, generally referred to as cruelty. There is obviously an implication here that sometimes suffering is necessary, or perhaps unavoidable, and so is not regarded as cruel. It is important, therefore, that we articulate and can explain exactly what we mean when we conclude that an animal is suffering; how have we reached that conclusion, are we being consistent and logical, have we considered what matters to the animal and not just what matters to us?

THE BEGINNING OF CONCERN FOR ANIMAL WELFARE

The British like to regard themselves as a 'nation of animal lovers'. This has not always been their reputation. In the eighteenth century many regarded England as the cruellest nation in Europe. Foreign visitors were shocked by the type and extent of practices involving animals regularly performed by all classes of people. Many of the pastimes now or recently carried out in other countries, and regarded as unacceptable by today's British public, such as bull running, (where bulls are run through a town until exhausted and then set upon by dogs or thrown off a bridge), and goose pulling, (where horsemen attempt to pull off the heads of live greased geese suspended upside down), were regularly performed for sport in Britain. Bull- and bear-baiting by dogs were common, as were all types of animal fighting, usually to the death. Cats were eaten alive at country fairs, cocks were tied to stakes and had sticks and stones thrown at them until they were dead, and schoolboys would bite the heads off sparrows, tie cats together by the tail and club hamstrung sheep to death.[4] Horses and dogs were used as draught animals and would regularly be subjected to excessively heavy workloads, beatings and mutilations.[5] Vast numbers of animals were killed for food, with many of them driven long distances into cities without food or water and then slaughtered by a variety of inhumane methods.[5] Calves were hung up alive by their Achilles tendon, hooks stuck through their nostrils, and slowly bled to death. Pigs were beaten to death in an attempt to improve meat quality. Geese, with their eyes removed, were nailed to boards and force-fed.[4]

The attitudes of the majority towards animals at this time were based on a combination of beliefs: that 'brutes' (animals) were insensible and without feeling, that God had bestowed on man a divine right of dominion, and therefore the ability to use animals for whatever purpose he chose, and finally that animals were absolute property in law, and so could be used or disposed of in any way the owner saw fit, without any intervention by others, in the same way as inanimate objects. It is interesting how these beliefs, or elements of them, still underpin many people's attitudes to animals today, even though we might find their spoken assertion abhorrent or uncomfortable. René Descartes (1596–1650) was a French philosopher and mathematician who was influential in determining attitudes towards animals, particularly in scientific circles. Descartes believed that animals were simply machines, and any actions or behaviours they performed, which might appear to indicate feelings or consciousness, were no more significant than the action of a clock or automaton. Only humans had souls, and therefore only humans were conscious and sentient. An animal's cries or struggles could be safely ignored, according to this view, since they meant nothing and need not be regarded. Animals were 'things' and unable to suffer.

There were some who did not subscribe to this theory, or the ideas that God-given dominion or property rights permitted cruel treatment of animals. During the eighteenth century, a growing body of work was published by philosophers, poets and politicians, challenging the status quo. The challenge was not just in relation to animals, but to the way in which humans themselves were treated. It was during this period that the concept of human rights, including the rights of women and slaves, was beginning to be aired. In 1776 Dr Humphry Primatt wrote 'Pain is Pain, whether it be inflicted on man or on beast; and the creature that suffers it, whether man or beast, being sensible of the misery of it whilst it lasts, suffers Evil.'[6] He also made an analogy between racism and animal exploitation: 'The white man ... can have no right, by virtue of his colour, to enslave and tyrannise over a black man ... for the same reason, a man can have no natural right to abuse and torment a beast'.[6] Perhaps the most famous author of the time, in relation to the status of animals, was Jeremy Bentham (1748–1832), a philosopher who promoted the idea of utilitarianism. What he wrote in 1780 still has great resonance today for those campaigning for a more compassionate approach to animals, and a greater status for them in law.

> The day may come when the rest of the animal creation may acquire those rights which never could have been withheld from them but by the hand of tyranny ... a full-grown horse or dog is beyond comparison a more rational, as well as a more conversable animal, than an infant of a day, or a week or even a month old. But supposed the case were otherwise, what could it avail? The question is not, can they reason? Nor, can they talk? But *can they suffer?* Why should the law refuse its protection to any sensitive being? The time will come when humanity will extend its mantle over everything which breathes ...[7]

Interestingly, one element of the concern for some people about the cruel and violent treatment of animals was the view that such acts were linked to more widespread and divisive antisocial behaviour. The idea that those who treat animals cruelly are more likely to treat their fellow man inhumanely ways was common amongst those of an 'improving' nature. Unkindness to animals was therefore undesirable, not necessarily because of the effects on the animals themselves, but because of the desensitising and dehumanising effects on the perpetrator, a conclusion which is acknowledged in modern times through the link between human and animal abuse.[8]

There was a desire, then, amongst certain quarters at least, by the beginning of the nineteenth century to halt the worst atrocities of animal cruelty, particularly when carried out for mere human pleasure or caprice. The only way to bring this about was by using legislation.

THE FIRST LEGISLATION

The initial targets for legislation were those activities carried out by what were known as the lower social orders. Indeed, for the next two centuries, and into the present day, there would be argument and debate about the relationship between legitimate pursuits involving animals and social class. By the early 1800s, bull baiting was largely a pastime of the working classes, and had become associated with disorderly and immoral public conduct. It became, therefore, the focus for the first of several attempts to outlaw this type of practice, in part because of the suffering of the animal but also because of the perceived unfortunate effect on the behaviour of those who participated.

The first Bills to prohibit bull baiting and cruelty to animals, presented to Parliament during the early nineteenth century, were rejected. Many Members of Parliament felt that these were not appropriate or sufficiently important matters for government involvement, and that banning activities such as bull baiting would eventually lead to a restriction of upper class pursuits, like hunting and shooting. The man credited with successfully passing the first animal welfare legislation through parliament is Richard Martin (1754–1834), an MP for Galway with a reputation for flamboyancy, eccentricity, a quick temper and great kindness both to animals and his fellow man. He did not, however, work alone, and was helped substantially by others, such as Lord Erskine and John Lawrence, to produce a Bill in 1821 which was eventually passed by both Houses of Parliament (in 1822) and became known as 'Martin's Act'. The Act made it an offence for any person or persons (importantly including the owner) to wantonly and cruelly beat, abuse, or ill-treat any horse, mare, gelding, mule, ass, ox, cow, heifer, steer, sheep, or other cattle.[5] For the next four years, Martin tried unsuccessfully to extend legal protection to other domestic animals, and to ban cruel sports. He unfortunately then lost his parliamentary seat, and so was unable to continue with his legislative reforms.

THE ARRIVAL OF THE RSPCA

Martin also campaigned for animals outside Parliament. No recognisable police force existed at the time, and unless someone chose to bring a prosecution under Martin's Act before the magistrates, the law would remain unenforced and therefore useless. It was Martin himself who brought the first prosecutions. It is reported that he sought out perpetrators to bring before the court, and would then often ask for the minimum sentence to be imposed upon conviction and pay the fine himself.[5] His aim was not to punish individuals, but to raise awareness of the Act and the plight of animals in general, and also to establish some case law in the courts.

From this approach in 1822 was born a fledgling society, initially known as the Society for the Prevention of Cruelty to Animals (SPCA), with the purpose of securing 'the mitigation of animal suffering, and the promotion and expansion of the practice of humanity towards the inferior classes of animated beings', using a combination of education and enforcement.[5] Martin was amongst the first members of the Society, which included eminent MPs, clerics, journalists and well known humanitarians. During the early days of the SPCA it came perilously close to being dissolved due to financial difficulties, but the Society built on the early foundations laid by Martin and his influential contemporaries, to eventually become one of the most famous animal welfare societies in the world. Initial successes were the introduction of improved conditions at Smithfield meat market in London, veterinary treatment of animals belonging to the poor, and the employment of two 'inspectors' and 270 successful prosecutions in 1837.[5] But more crucial was the ability of the Society to lobby those in positions of power and bring about a series of improvements, expansions and acts of enforcement in the protection, provided by the law, to animals.

Perhaps one of the most important events in the fortunes of the SPCA was the awarding of royal patronage. Before she became queen, Princess Victoria agreed to become a patroness of the Society, and after her ascension to the throne, the SPCA was allowed, in 1840, to use the prefix 'Royal'. As the RSPCA, it was able to command greater respect and recognition, given the high regard in which the aristocracy and the Queen were held at the time, and many other worthy and well-bred ladies became involved in the cause. From this time, concern for the plight of animals came to be seen as a more feminine interest, and much of the criticism from those who opposed greater protection for animals centred round the perceived 'womanly' and overly sentimental nature of the concern. What should be remembered, however, is that the early reformists in the field of animal welfare were generally men, and men who were far from 'sissy' or effeminate. It is also important to recognise that any improvement in the fortunes of animals went hand in hand with, (albeit sometimes in advance of), improvements in the status of other oppressed and disregarded members of society, such as slaves, women and working class children.

VIVISECTION AND THE ROLE OF SCIENCE

The biggest welfare issue of the second half of the nineteenth century was vivisection; the dissection of living, and generally fully conscious animals. This practice, more commonly seen on the continent than in Britain, was carried out at the time for both scientific discovery and as a form of entertainment and spectacle. The detailed descriptions of the procedures endured by animals, particularly dogs, make harrowing reading today, and indeed were deeply offensive to those in the new animal welfare movement of the time.[4] The RSPCA was officially opposed to many of the methods employed by vivisectionists, who were usually physiologists and physicians, but was regarded by many as being weak and ineffectual in tackling the issue. Science, and scientists, were powerful and the RSPCA council was unwilling to condemn outright the practice of vivisection, when carried out in order to further scientific knowledge and potentially alleviate human suffering.

Frances Power Cobbe (1822–1904), a writer and social worker, became perhaps the most persistent and prolific anti-vivisection crusader of the time. She organised the first example of a coordinated campaign against animal experimentation using petitions or 'memorials' signed by long and impressive lists of influential members of the aristocracy, the church and the ruling classes. These were presented to the RSPCA and the press, and used to bring pressure on the Government. Frustrated by the lack of will in the RSPCA, she set up her own Victoria Street Society, and eventually the British Union for the Abolition of Vivisection (which still exists today) in order to lobby and submit Bills for the regulation of vivisection to Parliament. Queen Victoria again added her considerable influence to the welfare movement by making her opposition to the dissection of conscious animals known both to the RSPCA, to whom she sent a donation specifically for the purpose of their campaign, and to her somewhat apathetic government ministers. It is debatable whether any legislation would actually have been passed had she not taken such a personal interest.

Bills introduced by Cobbe to Parliament, with the aim of banning or at least limiting the use of live animals in research, were successfully blocked by the powerful scientific and medical community, who strongly resented any suggestion of regulation. Because of this controversy a Royal Commission was set up in 1875 to look into the issue, and it took evidence from a wide variety of people. It is striking that the evidence provided by some scientists to support their cause served to so horrify the members of the Commission that they concluded that a problem did indeed exist. One lecturer at St Bartholomew's Hospital stated so starkly how little regard he had for the suffering or feelings of his animal subjects, and demonstrated such a complete lack of any humanity, that those taking his evidence were shocked.[4] The Commission eventually concluded that the use of animals in research, when carried out for legitimate purposes, was not, in itself, immoral, but limits were required, and certain practices should be banned, such as the use of dissection merely for the acquisition of manual skills or demonstration. After much government fudging, the Cruelty to Animals Act 1876 was passed. This was nowhere near as strict

as Cobbe would have wished, but did introduce licensing for those engaged in research using animals, and established a Home Office Inspectorate. The Act required the use of anaesthetics and humane techniques where possible, but its success yet again depended on motivated enforcement and there were many ways for those in the field to operate outside, or in spite of, the law. The 1876 Act remained in place for more than one hundred years and was continuously the subject of proposed reform and controversy.

This period of debate regarding vivisection coincided with a general rise in the profile and importance of science. Scientists then, and often still now, were keen to separate science from any moral considerations, suggesting that it was a discipline apart, without value judgements, and so should not be constrained in any way. The undisputed benefits brought to mankind through science served to make it difficult for those opposed to some scientific practices to argue against them successfully. It is also worth noting that Charles Darwin, an enthusiastic supporter of science, also published his revolutionary ideas on evolution and the origins of man during this time. The full implications of his conclusions on the close relationship between ourselves and other animals were not fully appreciated at the time, and arguably have still not been to this day. While some scientists were arguing that animals could and should be used in science because they were unlike people, and outside moral concern, another particularly influential scientist, Charles Darwin, was arguing how much alike we are to animals, and this inevitably has huge consequences for our relationship with them.

THE PROTECTION OF ANIMALS ACT 1911 AND INTO THE PRESENT DAY

Legislation that was first introduced in 1822 (Martin's Act) was amended and added to over the years. Many proposals for change were not passed, but issues such as wild animals, the use of dogs as draught animals, the export of live horses, recognition of mental as well as physical suffering, stray dogs, pit ponies, animal traps and animal transportation were all addressed, some more successfully than others, by legislation.[9] In 1911 all this legislative activity was consolidated into a new Protection of Animals Act mainly due to the efforts of George Greenwood MP. The 1911 Act (Protection of Animals Act 1912 in Scotland) is still in force today (including its subsequent amendments) and is used as the basis for nearly all prosecutions in relation to suffering and cruelty in domestic and captive animals. The Government is currently in the process of drafting a new Bill to modernise and rationalise the existing animal welfare legislation, but many elements and ideas found in the 1911 Act will still be present in a new Bill, and so an understanding of its wording and origins is useful.

The Act makes it an offence if any person 'shall cruelly beat, kick, ill-treat, over-ride, over-drive, over-load, torture, infuriate, or terrify any animal, or shall cause or procure, or being the owner, permit any animal to be so used, or shall, by wantonly or unreasonably doing or omitting to do any act, or causing or procuring the commission or omission of any act, cause any unnecessary suffering, or, being the owner, permit any unnecessary suffering to be so caused to any domestic animal'. Previously banned or regulated activities are also included in the wording of the Act; fighting, baiting, poisoning, the performing of any operation without due care and attention, knackers' yards, the use of dogs for draught on public roads, the inspection of traps for catching hares and rabbits and the release of an animal in an injured, mutilated or exhausted condition for the purpose of hunting or coursing. Police officers are able to order the destruction of an injured animal on the advice of a veterinary surgeon. Courts are able to confiscate animals and are able to impose greater penalties upon conviction than previously.

Wording from the very early legislation can be seen in the 1911 Act, and when considering the situation of animals at the time, the cumbersome and old-fashioned terms used make more sense. Some important features of the Act need to be understood to explain the situation with regard to the legal status and protection of animals in the present day. Firstly, despite the Act being called the Protection of Animals Act, animals must in fact suffer before an offence is committed, and so are often offered precious little *protection* from suffering. Enforcement bodies are, therefore, powerless

to intervene, even when they can see that an animal is about to suffer, whether through neglect or direct infliction of cruelty. They must wait until the event has taken place and the unfortunate animal has suffered the abuse. Secondly, it must be established that the suffering was not necessary. It would clearly not be appropriate for someone who unintentionally injures an animal by hitting it with their car, for example, to be prosecuted in the same way as someone who causes a similar injury because of recklessness or vicious intent. Generally speaking 'unnecessary suffering' is suffering which is disproportionate to what the person is trying to achieve, which is not inevitable, and could have been avoided or terminated. So, making an animal suffer just to make life flow more comfortably or to save money, for instance, would not be acceptable. Thirdly, the court must decide in each case whether a reasonably competent, reasonably humane person would have done the same thing in the circumstances. It is not necessary to prove that the person committing the offence meant to be cruel, otherwise stupid and ignorant people would always have a defence, but the measure is whether a 'reasonable' person should have known that an animal was being caused to suffer.

Another important feature of the current legal situation is the continued status of animals as property, rather than beings with any defined rights or privileges. Albeit that the infliction of suffering on an animal is prohibited, the owner still commands total control over the destiny and purpose of that animal's life. If an owner wishes to use an animal in a particular way, including the killing of that animal, they have complete discretion to do so within the limits described above. This has certain practical advantages and disadvantages, and a profound effect on any ethical debate about the possibility of animals possessing any inherent rights within society. One advantage is that if an animal has an owner, that person can then be identified and obliged by law to care and provide for it during the time they are deemed to own it. Otherwise, who would be responsible for providing for an animal's needs – the State, the local community, the animal itself? Disadvantages are experienced when owners use their animals in ways which others find morally repugnant, the performing of tricks for entertainment and profit, or for the mass production of food or fur, for example.

The immense and profound events of the First and Second World Wars effectively halted any further significant progress in the fields of improved legal protection and promotion of animal interests. There were no serious attempts to improve or update the 1911 Act until the beginning of the twenty first century. Philosophers began to take a serious interest in animals again, and their particular issues within society, during the 1960s and 70s, with the publication of work by authors such as Ruth Harrison (who highlighted the plight of animals in the new 'factory' farms). Peter Singer published 'Animal Liberation' and described in graphic detail the unfair and unjustified treatment of animals by man, and Tom Regan argued for the recognition of animals' inherent worth and rights as sentient beings.

ANIMAL WELFARE PROTECTION TODAY

The Protection of Animals Act 1911 is unusual in that it is enforced almost exclusively by the RSPCA, a charitable organisation with no legal standing in its own right, and funded entirely by voluntary donation. The Society has a team of uniformed inspectors as its public face of enforcement, but they have no powers of search or entry beyond that of any other citizen. Although they are trained to operate using legally acceptable standards of evidence-gathering, they are reliant upon police officers to actually enforce the Act, in relation to seizure of animals and entry into private premises. In 2003, the RSPCA employed 323 inspectors and achieved 1829 convictions for cruelty, with a total cost (of the Inspectorate, prosecutions and operations) of £36,434,000.[10] The unique role of the RSPCA has arisen because it has been involved in both lobbying to introduce legislation, and then using the legislation to prosecute offenders, with the aim of protecting individual animals and raising the profile of animal welfare, for such a long time. No recognisable police force was in existence when Richard Martin began his campaign of test cases to create awareness of his new Act, and the RSPCA has assumed responsibility for animal welfare in the eyes of the public and government enforcement bodies. This has the advantage for the RSPCA that it is able to choose which cases it brings to court, on the basis of benefit for the animals concerned, and perhaps more importantly, on the basis of making a public statement of acceptable standards, rather than just on the realistic chances of a successful prosecution. High public awareness of the RSPCA means it is able to exert a considerable level of influence for a charitable body, but it sometimes appears to be viewed by many as another branch of social services, with statutory responsibility for animal welfare matters. Local authorities and the State Veterinary Service do have responsibility for enforcing some animal welfare legislation, but tend to be fundamentally under-resourced and have other, sometimes more pressing, demands on their time and funds. The police have stated their own unwillingness to assume responsibility for animal welfare enforcement.[11]

The role of the European Union (initially known as the European Community) should not be ignored when looking at the regulation of animal welfare. In 1999 (through the Treaty of Amsterdam) the original founding treaty of the European Community was extended to include a clause stating that animals were sentient beings, and that both the EU and Member States must pay full regard to this, when formulating or implementing their policies. Prior to this, live animals in EC law were simply categorised as agricultural products and so were subject to the same rules of trade as potatoes or sugar. A great raft of legislation concerned with the welfare of farmed animals has been issued from Brussels since the 1980s, culminating in the acknowledgement of their unique status (albeit an inadequate acknowledgement for some) within the founding treaty of the Union. Progress is slow but the battery cage for laying hens will be banned throughout the EU by 2012, the permanent tethering of sows will be banned in 2006 and the use of stalls (where sows are unable to walk or turn around) for pregnant sows, beyond four weeks gestation, will be prohibited after 2013. Minimum standards for animals on farm, during transport and at the time of slaughter are in place across all countries of the EU and this must be regarded as a welcome step and provides, at the least, a mechanism for further improvement.

Two of the most significant shortcomings of current animal welfare legislation are the lack of actual pre-emptive protection provided to animals under the 1911 Act, and the fact that animals will often be given different levels of protection depending on what type of animal they are, and where they happen to be at the time. There is extensive and sometimes detailed legislation for some types of commercial farm animal but scant and very general requirements for dogs, for example, unless they happen to be held in a designated research establishment. Since 1911, there have been so many amendments and additions to welfare law that the area can be complicated, complex and inconsistent. Certain activities involving animals require a licence, such as selling animals in a pet shop, keeping a riding school or operating a zoo, but the requirements necessary to achieve a licence range from the most rudimentary administrative details to an annual visit from an expert in the field. What is needed is a revamping and reorganisation of all existing animal welfare law and the introduction of a more uniform approach so that the overall aim of society, to provide a degree of protection to the animals affected by it, can be achieved in practice.

This is the purpose of the proposed new Animal Welfare Bill. The Bill will have broad and general principles designed to reflect a modern attitude towards animals and all existing welfare legislation (except the Animals (Scientific Procedures) Act 1986 which covers animals used in research) will be brought under its umbrella. It will also provide a mechanism for future legislation to be passed which will reflect the changing status of animals over the next century. The offence of cruelty or causing unnecessary suffering will probably remain much the same, along with the offence of staging animal fights. A crucial new addition is likely to be a requirement to positively promote an animal's welfare rather than just not inflict suffering. The proposal is a new offence of failure to take reasonable steps to ensure an animal's welfare. What precisely is covered by the term welfare, and how this is to be determined, are not defined, but the proposed assessment is based around the Five Freedoms (freedom from hunger and thirst; freedom from discomfort; freedom from pain, injury and disease; freedom from fear and distress and freedom to express normal behaviour) which are commonly used in the farm animal context.[12]

THE VETERINARY PROFESSION

The role of the veterinary profession in the history of animal welfare might have appeared noticeably absent during the earlier part of this chapter. Veterinary surgeons are considered, in law and by the majority of the public, to be experts in the field of welfare, but have in fact become involved in the subject relatively late in the day. The first origins of the profession were relatively humble, with most so-called practitioners having no training and relying on idiosyncratic and unproven 'cures' which are unlikely to have done much to help their patients. The first records of veterinary training date from 1791 when a private college was established in London, with another school opening in Edinburgh during the 1820s. The reputation of veterinary science, however, did not achieve any great status until the end of the nineteenth century, when the passing of formal examinations was required before participants were allowed to use the title 'veterinary surgeon' and were entitled to become registered members of the Royal College of Veterinary Surgeons (RCVS).[9] For many years the RCVS was unable to prevent untrained or unregistered people from misleadingly holding themselves out as veterinary surgeons, a situation which served to jeopardise the reputation of the fledgling profession, but by 1881 it became an offence to falsely hold oneself out as a registered veterinary surgeon. Further veterinary schools were founded at Glasgow, Liverpool and Dublin and later at Cambridge and Bristol and the standing and reputation of the profession has increased significantly in recent years.

The earliest records of the veterinary nursing profession date back to the beginning of the 1900s, when the first small animal hospitals and nursing homes were established. The Canine Nurses Institute was set up in 1908 by a Mrs Lenty Collins, and uniformed nurses were trained in the care of dogs and the proper conduct of a nurse. Other centres were established over the years to provide health care for sick small animals, and these would commonly include the attentions of veterinary nurses. In 1961, the RCVS started the first veterinary nursing qualifications with the establishment of Registered Animal Nursing Auxiliaries or RANA, the term 'nurse' being protected at the time for those in the human field. Qualified Veterinary Nurses appeared in 1984.[13]

On the whole, the veterinary profession has responded to society's expectations and attitudes towards animals rather than shaped them. Vets, as a body, have been reluctant to become involved in campaigns over controversial welfare issues such as animal experimentation, blood sports and intensive farming. An influential philosopher, Richard Ryder, is of the opinion that although 'widely seen by members of the public as being interested in the welfare of animals, with a few glorious exceptions, vets have been distinguished by their absence from the great campaigns of the last two hundred years'.[14] He also asserts that the vested interests of members of the profession have prevented their publicly criticising certain practices. There is an inherent tension in the role of a veterinary surgeon, in that they must act on behalf of their client, but also swear an oath that their 'constant endeavour will be to ensure the welfare of animals committed to my care'.[15] Where vets are required to work in situations with potential for the compromise of animal welfare, their role as either servant or animal advocate often remains undefined and needs further exploration, both by the profession and those who rely on its services. In recent years, the profession has assumed a greater role in the formation of opinion and policy with the issuing of more detailed guidance to its members, and statements of policy, in relation to tail docking in dogs and renal transplantation in cats, for example.

CONCLUSION

This chapter has outlined the historical context of the current animal welfare situation. An understanding of this background is important to explain our somewhat complicated legal system in relation to animals, and many of our apparent inconsistencies as a society. When reviewing past campaigns for change, and the debates which raged at the time, is it interesting to note how many of the issues and opinions are still relevant today. There is still heartfelt and determined opposition to experimentation and research involving animals, and the matter of hunting with dogs still raises questions about class and the nature of a legitimate pursuit. In many respects we have moved on significantly since the days when animals were casually and brutally ill-used as a matter of routine or principle, but there are new challenges for those wishing to improve the lot of animals. Intensive farming practices, endangered wild animals and the effects of increased global trade are all arguably causing worsening problems for animals and the solutions are not within easy reach. Within the veterinary world, the advent of more advanced treatments and techniques raises questions of how much intervention can be justified to keep animals alive, and the gap between the treatment received by animals of certain species, belonging to affluent owners, and less favoured animals in commercial situations, often hidden from public view, is ever widening.

References

1. Broom DM, Johnson KG. Stress and animal welfare. The Netherlands: Kluwer; 1993:75–82.
2. Dawkins MS. Behavioural deprivation: a central problem in animal welfare. Applied Animal Behaviour Science 1988; 20:209–225.
3. Duncan IJH. Welfare is to do with what animals feel. Journal of Agricultural and Environmental Ethics 1993; 6 (supplement 2):8–14.
4. Ryder RD. Animal revolution. Oxford: Berg; 2000.
5. Radford M. Animal welfare law in Britain: regulation and responsibility. Oxford: Oxford University Press: 2001:39–43.
6. Primatt H. The duty of mercy and the sin of cruelty to brute animals. London 1776:14–18. In: Ryder RD, ed. Animal revolution. Oxford: Berg; 2000:62.

7. Bentham J. Introduction to the principles of morals and legislation. 1780:Ch 17. In: Ryder RD, ed. Animal revolution. Oxford: Berg; 2000:71.

8. RCVS issues guidelines on dealing with abuse in animals and humans. Veterinary Record 2003; 152(15):446–447.

9. Radford M. Animal welfare law in Britain: regulation and responsibility. Oxford: Oxford University Press: 2001:Chs 3–4.

10. RSPCA Annual Review 2003. Online. Available: http://www.rspca.org.uk 9 May 2005.

11. DEFRA. Consultation on an Animal Welfare Bill – An analysis of the replies. August 2002:152. Online. Available: http://www.defra.gov.uk/animalh/welfare/bill/index.htm 10 October 2005.

12. Farm Animal Welfare Council. FAWC updates the five freedoms. Veterinary Record 1992; 131:357.

13. Turner J. The evolution of veterinary nursing. Veterinary Nursing Journal 1994; 9:103–108.

14. Ryder RD. Animal revolution. Oxford: Berg; 2000:190.

15. Royal College of Veterinary Surgeons. Guide to professional conduct: Introduction. Online. Available: http://www.rcvs.org.uk 9 May 2005.

Further reading

Appleby MC. What should we do about animal welfare? Oxford: Blackwell Science: 1999.

Radford M. Animal welfare law in Britain. Oxford: Oxford University Press: 2001.

Ryder R. Animal revolution. Oxford: Berg: 2000.

Spedding C. Animal Welfare. London: Earthscan; 2000.

Webster J. Animal welfare – a cool eye towards Eden. Oxford: Blackwell Science: 1994.

7

Religious ethics

Giles Legood

In this chapter we shall consider how much of the current interest in human treatment of animals has been informed by religious conviction. We will also note that human action on animals has, in starkly different ways, been motivated by religious belief for centuries, indeed millennia. In doing so it will be both necessary and useful to look at how the major religious traditions currently found in Britain broadly regard animals. Such an understanding not only helps us become better citizens by understanding more fully what motivates those around us, but will also help readers to become better veterinary nurses since, as we shall see, the religious beliefs of human beings affect the treatment of both domestic and non-domestic animals committed to their care.

Any person who takes even the most cursory look at the newspapers, or who only occasionally listens to the radio or watches the television news cannot fail to notice that the reporting and discussion of human treatment of animals is both newsworthy and of great public interest. It is certainly true to say that each day, in the national media, there is an item which involves ethical or welfare issues concerning animals. Such issues typically include hunting, genetic engineering, laboratory animals, veal crates, whaling, the wearing of fur, dog fighting, puppy farms, badger baiting, stray dogs, fishing, intensive poultry farming, transportation, exotic pets, zoos and circuses. This interest is no new phenomenon; there is an extremely long history of debate and disagreement as to what we may legitimately do to non-human animals and what our duties and responsibilities are towards them. All of these issues, and others related to

them, will be of interest to the veterinary nurse, both professionally and personally.

ANCIENT PHILOSOPHY

For centuries, philosophers did not defend the moral status of animals very seriously. For instance, the philosopher Pythagoras (*c.* 570 BC) and his followers did show some care for animals, not because such action was good in itself, but only on the basis that when eating some cooked meat, they might be inadvertently eating the implanted soul of an ancestor. This was their belief in the doctrine of metempsychosis, where the souls of the dead may enter not only bodies of humans but also of animals. Pythagoras is reported to have tried to prevent someone from whipping a puppy because when he heard it bark he recognised the voice of a departed friend.

Many see Aristotle (384–322 BC) as being responsible for the superior attitude adopted by many in the West towards animals. Aristotle held that only those who were rational, that is, had the power of reason, were entitled to special moral status. Animals, he believed, were without reason and therefore humankind had no responsibilities or duties towards them. In his work *Politics* he writes 'Since nature makes nothing without some end in view, nothing to no purpose, it must be that nature has made animals and plants for the sake of humans.' This view endured for centuries and indeed is still held by many today. Two thousand years after Aristotle wrote those words, Nicholas Fontaine in 1738 observed a practical working-out of such a view: 'They administered beatings to dogs with perfect indifference and made fun of those who pitied the creatures as if they felt pain . . . They nailed poor animals up on boards by their paws to vivisect them and see the circulation of the blood, which was a great subject of conversation'.[1]

Although Plato and Aristotle held conventional religious views for their day (Aristotle gave theology the highest rank in possible studies), neither might easily be regarded as 'religious' thinkers. Their views of God were to regard God as the Unmoved Mover, a metaphysical principle which did not make demands on daily human living but which rather was concerned with how the world was made and how it operated physically. More formal, prescribed belief systems, where religion has implications for human behaviour which we might recognise, would have been unknown to them.

RELIGIOUS ATTITUDES

In the last century, archaeological work showed us that, as far as we can tell, Neanderthal humans, living 150,000 years ago, were intensely religious in their outlook. Despite the claims made by adherents of secularism, religions have been and, for the majority of the world's population, still are major forces in human life. In thinking through issues surrounding both the ethics and the history of animal welfare, the influence of religion cannot be ignored for it has motivated many of those working in the field of animal welfare and thus underlies and informs many of the theories and discussions around the issues of the human use of animals. Indeed, it has motivated also those who have not thought of themselves as working in the sphere of animal welfare but who have, nevertheless, simply by their everyday interaction with animals, had this action informed by religious belief. Of course, such belief need not even overtly influence human action but its pull has been strong, just the same.

Religious beliefs may raise questions about how consensus can be reached in disagreement relating to how animals should be treated. While what we might call 'humane' treatment of animals may well be motivated by religious belief, it is equally

the case that 'inhumane' treatment might also arise from religious conviction. Where human uses and abuses of animals take place from religious conviction, it is likely that discussion as to why an action has been taken might not go beyond 'Because God/scripture says it is so'. Indeed, simply to talk of 'abuses' of animals is question-begging since it presumes a position which is held by the person using the term and is, in itself, open for argument. In the world of veterinary science, where scientific enquiry is the usual discourse, metaphysical claims relating to God/scripture (that is, claims which cannot be tested by experience or observation) may not sit easily. Nevertheless, to understand something of the motivations and beliefs of others is important, both in recognition that we are all different and to help engender a greater empathy amongst us all. Better understanding of clients and their animals makes for better veterinary nursing and veterinary nurses.

WORLD RELIGIONS

The following is a brief introduction to the main beliefs of some of the world's major religions and their attitudes towards animals. For the first time, in 2001, the national household census of the United Kingdom asked those completing the census forms to fill out a voluntary question on religious affiliation. The first five religions listed below were the five religions with the most adherents in Britain (and indeed in the world). In addition to these, brief mention is also made of Jainism and the Baha'i faith as these two religions have significant views on human behaviour towards animals. Followers of other religions were, of course, found by the survey but, given the small numbers involved, it is unlikely that the veterinary nurse will come across many owners whose treatment of their animals has been motivated by these minority beliefs.

Judaism

Although there are only 17 million Jews in the world, adherents of this religion have had an enormous influence on world history. Not only has Judaism provided some of the world's greatest thinkers – Moses, Jesus, Freud, Einstein – it also provided the religious outlook from which Christianity emerged. Jews believe there is one God, a God who has a covenant relationship with the Jewish people. God's requirements of his people are set out in the *Torah* (what Christians regard as the first five books of the Old Testament) and holiness is obtained by observing its teaching. Jews believe that God acts through history and that in the future God will vindicate his promises through the coming of a Messiah. Many of the teachings of Judaism emphasise kindness towards animals and a general reverence towards nature. Jewish law is strict in its requirement that animals be treated properly. It demands that close attention is paid to pets and domestic animals, indeed the *Talmud* (the source of oral law, coming from the Rabbis) states that people must provide for their animals before they themselves sit down to eat or drink. It also states that an animal should not be kept unless it can be cared for and fed. Mediaeval Rabbis spoke of the obligation to provide for homeless animals; beasts of burden should not be overloaded, nor should cats and dogs be tormented. Jewish law disapproves of hunting and other blood sports and one of the Ten Commandments requires that animals be allowed to rest on the Sabbath. The part of the tradition concerning animals, which is perhaps regarded as the most controversial today, is that of *kosher* killing (kosher is a Hebrew word meaning 'Fit for use'). These rituals were originally prescribed in order to minimise animal pain and suffering but are thought by many to be inhumane. The method of ritual slaughter (*schechitah*) requires that an animal should have its throat cut by a very sharp knife, without any pre-stunning. Some Jews, and others, feel that more modern methods of killing should now be used and that this would be in keeping with the original spirit of the law.

Christianity

Christianity is the religion of the followers of Jesus, a Palestinian Jew who lived approximately 2000 years ago. Christians believe that this Jesus was the Son of God, sent by God to re-establish the broken link between humankind and God. In this way, Jesus is regarded as the Messiah who has overcome the human tendency towards selfishness by living a selfless life and finally dying as an innocent victim on a cross. Scripture, tradition and reason are given weight within Christianity. Christian scriptures (the Bible) consist of the Jewish texts, written before Jesus (the Old Testament) and texts written some decades after the life of Jesus (the New Testament). The Jewish texts have a strong theme of kindness towards animals. In the first book of the Bible, God gives humankind dominion over the creatures of the earth. This dominion is a stewardship, which brings responsibilities and duties towards animals and the rest of the natural world. The New Testament has many references to Jesus entreating his followers to protect animals. Jesus uses animal imagery to illustrate his teaching and teaches that God loves even the smallest of creatures, 'Are not two sparrows sold for two pennies? And not one of them is forgotten before God.' Many of the saints of the Christian church are said to have had a close and loving relationship with animals. St Francis of Assisi (1181–1226) called the animals his 'brothers and sisters'. Other Christians, however, reflected the Aristotelian tradition of disregarding animals as having much worth, because they lacked rational souls. Where kindness towards animals was commended it was often only because it was believed that such acts would predispose humans to be kinder towards one another. Such was the attitude of many in the West for centuries, because for this time Christianity was the dominant, or only, religion represented in the population. An increasing number of contemporary Christians are returning to the example of St Francis, and today a number of churches have prayers and services for, or in celebration of, animals.

Buddhism

Buddhism contains many different forms of belief and organisation and cannot properly be called a single religion, rather it is a family of religions. Buddhism was founded by Siddartha Gautama (566–486 BC) who, after entering a grove and meditating, experienced the ecstasy of *Nirvana* – the losing of greed, hatred and delusion. From this point on Gautama became known as the Buddha (the Enlightened One). In the *Dharma* (the teaching) the Buddha tells us that all life forms are interrelated and part of a larger unified life force. Thus, to do harm to any part of this single entity is to harm oneself and all life. One of the injunctions of Buddhist monks and lay associates is 'Refrain from destroying life' (*ahimsa*). The Dharma states 'Whoever in seeking happiness inflicts pain on beings which also seek happiness, shall find no happiness after death'. Buddhist teaching frowns on the eating of meat, the killing of animals for sport, the selling of land where animals may be hunted or killed and the use of animals in medical research. Buddhists may not provide for others anything, such as nets, weapons and poisons, which may be used to inflict injury on other living beings. Indeed the Dharma states that humans 'must not hate any being and cannot kill a living creature even in thought'.

Islam

Islam is the fastest growing major religion in the world and has been responsible for one of the truly great civilisations of the world. Islam holds that there is one God (*Allah*) and that idolatry and polytheism are mistaken. Muhammad (born 570 AD) is regarded as the Prophet of God, to whom God has given absolute and final revelation. The revelation is contained in the *Qur'an*. Muslims are required to observe the Five Pillars of Islam: witnessing to the faith; ritual prayer; fasting during the month of Ramadan; charity; pilgrimage to Mecca. Islam has very strict prohibitions against cruelty to animals. The scripture called the Hadith contains the traditions of the Prophet. The Hadith tells us that 'all creatures are like a family of God; and He loves the most those who are the most beneficent to His family'. Muhammad often spoke of the rewards and punishments which individuals would receive on Judgement Day, according to their treatment of animals. He also spoke of 'Kill not a living creature, which Allah has made sacrosanct, except for justifiable reason'. The Prophet also condemned blood sports, inciting animals to fight and the trading of wild animal pelts. Islam sets clear limits as to what is or is not permissible in regard to animals. Animals may be used for food, clothing, as beasts of burden and as a sacrifice in submission to Allah, although unnecessary abuse, overwork or cruelty to animals is forbidden. Islam places strong emphasis on food being halal (Arabic for 'That which is permitted'). Halal slaughter must be carried out by an approved pious Muslim of sound mind; the act must be done manually using a stainless steel knife which must be cleaned after each kill; the animal's respiratory tract, oesophagus, and jugular vein must be severed, and the animal must be dead before skinning takes place. Halal killing is exempt from the UK legislation which requires that animals be stunned prior to slaughter.

Hinduism

The term 'Hinduism' is something of a misnomer. It is a term which is convenient European shorthand for many of the varied religions of India, which are based on the ancient and sacred scriptures called the *Vedas* (written in approximately 1200 BC). To make generalisations can be misleading but the following beliefs are shared by most of those whom we might term 'Hindu'. The universe is interconnected across time and space. Rocks, plants, animals and humans are all interrelated and all are thought to have kinship with one another and to be worthy of respect and life. People are re-born and the location of the soul and body are determined by *karma* (the moral law of cause and effect where one's future existence is determined by the thoughts and actions of the present life). Hinduism therefore compels kindness to animals so as to aid re-incarnation (samsara) and because humans and animals are part of the same family. Many Hindu texts teach that all species should be treated as children. The cow has a special place in Hinduism, so much so that Gandhi said 'Protection of the cow means protection of the whole dumb creation of God'. Although many Hindus keep a vegetarian diet, others do eat meat. Some of the Hindu castes permit animal sacrifice and others would, under certain circumstances, allow animals to be used for scientific research if there were no alternatives and if it was clearly shown to result in human benefit.

Baha'ism

The Baha'i faith started as a development of the *Shiite* branch of Islam in Persia (modern day Iran), where today it is outlawed and considered a heresy. The founder of the faith, Baha'u'llah (translated as Glory of God, 1817–1892), taught that all religions should unite since the human race is one under God. Animals and the rest of the natural world are regarded as part of the unity of the earth and the universe.

Nature is held in high regard in the Baha'i faith, and there is a strong tradition of a love for, and a need to connect with, nature and the countryside. The founder's son and successor, Abdu'l-Baha (1844–1921) taught that humans occupy a position higher than the rest of nature, which they rule over, but that the natural world should be accorded respect. As part of this, compassionate treatment for animals is a basic tenet of Baha'ism and humans are required to show kindness towards animals. Indeed, tenderness and loving kindness to every living creature are regarded as basic principles of God's heavenly Kingdom. Abdu'l-Baha also taught that children should be taught to be tender towards animals from the earliest age. While meat eating is not prohibited it is strongly discouraged in the writings of the faith, since, the teaching says, even without meat humans would live with the 'utmost vigour and energy'.

Jainism

Of all of the world's religions, it would seem that Jainism is the most rigorous in efforts to avoid harming any living creature. In India, where most Jains live, monks of this religion sweep the path before them to avoid walking on insects. Other activities, designed to protect animals, include a refusal to turn over soil or to brew drinks, as this may harm mould, yeast and other lower forms of life.

Jainism was founded in India in the sixth century BC as an offshoot of Hinduism. Jainism sprung up as a reaction again the rigid caste system, especially that of the Brahmins (the priestly caste) and their claims of social and spiritual supremacy. The religion's founder, Mahavira, grew up in great luxury, but at the age of thirty he renounced all this, together with his wife and child, and became a monk. Following their founder, all Jains go to considerable lengths to avoid harm to animals. Some Jains wear masks over their mouths so as not to inhale tiny insects. They may also inspect all fruit before eating it to ensure that no small creature will be ingested. Some may only eat during the daytime, least small creatures be harmed inadvertently in the poor light of night. Most of these practices would only be carried out by Jain monks, whereas lay Jains might simply avoid eating meat, and never knowingly take a life or harm a sentient creature.

There are nearly four million Jains living in modern India. They fund and run a very large number of animal sanctuaries, where large animals such as cows, camels and water buffalo, as well as smaller animals such as pigeons and parrots, are cared for. The religious philosophy of these places seems to be that the spark of life is no dimmer simply because it is encased in fur or feather. Jainism, in its desire never to harm another living creature does take an absolutist stance on pain. If, for example, a bird with a broken wing is brought to one of the sanctuaries, those working there will not tend to the animal by giving it an injection to ease its pain, since this would involve harming the animal with a needle. Similarly, its wing could not be re-set since this would be interfering with the natural order of things and might also involve some discomfort to the animal.

RELIGION, ETHICS AND CULTURE

So far, in this chapter's consideration of religion and ethics, we have seen how ancient and religious views of animals have informed the thinking of our own culture and context. It is important for us to acknowledge that such discussions are not simply dispassionate observations, but part of the process whereby we are able to make sense of history, by understanding it better, and thus allow it to inform our present and future. Moral theory has a long, distinguished history and has developed a particular vocabulary in its striving to make itself both clear and open to further discussion. The word 'ethics' comes from the Greek word *ethicos* which in the plural means 'manners' or 'customs'. Ethics are then culture bound and what one society may feel is acceptable may be regarded as beyond the pale in another. Likewise, if viewed as what is customarily acceptable, ethics will differ from age to age. What is regarded as ethical, whether motivated by religious feeling or otherwise, in the twenty-first century may well have been viewed as immoral centuries before, and vice versa. Religious convictions, even those labelled by religious believers as 'truths', shift from time to time, according to culture and context, in the same way that morality does.

ANIMAL WELFARE AND RELIGIOUS CONVICTION

Britain is traditionally seen as a nation of animal lovers. Much of the change that has taken place over the last two hundred years, in terms of ethical thinking and legislation, has come about either because it has been motivated by religious conviction of individual reformers or because, until recently, Britain could be called a Christian country and its legal system and parliament were broadly framed by teachings of the Church. Eighteenth-century Britain, when legislative changes first came about, was a country in which calls for social reform arose and gained influential support. Parliament was unable to ignore the calls for radical social change which many notable individuals, often with a single issue as an aim, had been proclaiming. William Wilberforce's tireless work for the abolition of slavery finally succeeded in amending the law in 1807 after more than twenty years of campaigning. Other legislation aimed at outlawing, for instance, cruelty to children, also achieved success. Many of those who campaigned for such changes were motivated by a Christian conviction that it was an affront to the God who was made known in the person of Jesus that human beings, made in the image of God and all equally loved, should be treated so shamefully. It also occurred to many that this Christian concern for God's creation should include those non-human creatures, who were also created and loved by the same God. John Wesley (1703–1791), a Church of England priest and the founder of the movement which became known as Methodism, was a vegetarian and argued that humans had a duty to be tender towards animals because both humans and animals 'were the offspring of one common father'. Wesley's widespread preaching (he travelled 250,000

miles on horseback during his lifetime) and the writings of such people as Bishop Joseph Butler (1692–1752), had considerable influence on the change of attitude towards animals at this time.

It would be wrong however to think that only those inspired by religious allegiance were calling for changes of attitude and practice. One of the most influential campaigners for fairer treatment of animals was the economist and philosopher Jeremy Bentham. As previously mentioned, Bentham is best known for advocating, with JS Mill, the idea of utilitarianism. When faced with deciding which possible action to take, utilitarianism offers a simple equation for helping to decide. Simply expressed, according to Bentham, one should ask which action is going to bring about 'the greatest happiness for the greatest number' and pursue this. While Bentham took this equation to mean what will bring about the greatest *human* happiness, a number of philosophers have subsequently widened the scope of the equation to embrace animals too.

Towards the end of the eighteenth century two cases of animal cruelty came to public attention. These became instrumental in influencing public opinion to such an extent that there were widespread calls for law reform. In 1790, a man was unsuccessfully prosecuted for ripping out a horse's tongue whilst simultaneously beating it on the head. He was acquitted because there were no laws on the statute books at that time which gave any protection to animals from cruelty. In 1793, two butchers in Manchester were fined for cutting off the feet of live sheep and then driving the animals through the streets. The public was outraged, for not only had cruelty clearly taken place, but had the butchers owned the sheep themselves they could not have been prosecuted. At that time there was no legislation in place which prohibited cruelty towards an animal by its owner, and thus prosecution in such cases would only be successful on the grounds that a cruel act towards an animal had harmed someone else's property.

With such cases seizing the public imagination, legislation, or at least attempts at it, followed. In 1800 Sir William Pultney brought a Bill before Parliament to outlaw bull baiting. The Bill failed, as did a similar one two years later. Even at this stage the welfare of the animals was perhaps not paramount, as one of the arguments against the Bills was that 'it would be wrong to deprive the lower orders of their amusements'. Attempts at successfully introducing legislation continued, however, and in 1809, the Lord Chancellor, Thomas Erskine, introduced a Bill 'Preventing the Wanton and Malicious Cruelty Towards Animals'. Erskine's Bill was passed by the House of Lords but it failed in the Commons. Nevertheless supporters of laws to protect animals took heart that if such influential people as the Lord Chancellor were concerned about the matter, then the tide must be turning in their favour.

The date which is singularly most important in the history of animal welfare legislation in Britain is 22 July 1822. This is the date of the enactment of the first piece of legislation, known as 'Martin's Act', which gave protection to at least some categories of animals (see Chapter 6).

Although the argument in Parliament may have been won, cruelties, nevertheless, continued. It was still not uncommon for cat skinners to practise their trade. Here, the skins of cats were removed while the animals were still alive and then the animals were often thrown into the street. A number of people also made their living by stealing cats in order to provide the skinners with potential pelts. Pigs were routinely whipped to tenderise their flesh, shopkeepers kept squirrels in cages, running on treadmills, in order to attract customers and animals were taught to perform tricks for people's amusement through acts of torture and deprivation.

We noted earlier in the chapter that some of those most influential in campaigning for animal welfare legislation had also previously worked for improved conditions for humans who lived and worked in misery (notably as slaves or as child labour). At the time that Martin's Act was beginning to have an effect on the living conditions and treatment of animals, an organisation was founded by an Anglican priest, the Reverend Arthur Broome, to educate the public in the matter of humane treatment of animals. The first meeting of this 'Society for the Prevention of Cruelty to Animals' (the SPCA, later to become the RSPCA) was held in the appropriately named Old Slaughter's Coffee-House in St. Martin's Lane, London in 1824. Its first Secretary was John Colam, also Secretary of the National Society for the Prevention of Cruelty to Children, and one of its founding members was the prominent Christian Member of Parliament and anti-slavery leader, William Wilberforce.

These then were the changes in attitude and legislation up to mid-nineteenth century Britain, but perhaps the greatest influence on the treatment of animals came about through the scientific work of Charles Darwin (1809–82), the son of a clergyman. Although not the first person to put forward a theory of evolution by natural selection, Darwin was to see his theory gain wide acceptance both within the scientific community and wider society. In his two most notable publications, *The Origin of Species by Means of Natural Selection* (1859) and *The Descent of Man* (1871), Darwin blew apart the almost universally accepted theory that human beings were set apart biologically from the rest of the natural order. His views were widely disputed and opposed when he first published them, but Darwin's influence now means that human beings cannot easily believe themselves to be entirely separate from all other living organisms on the earth. Twenty years before *The Origin of Species* was published, Darwin put his view thus, 'Man in his arrogance thinks himself a great work worthy the interposition of a deity. More humble and I think truer to consider him created from animals'.[2]

It is not surprising, given his lifelong work of understanding the links between human beings and animals, that Darwin was also one of those who worked hard to promote the introduction of the 1876 Cruelty to Animals Act. This Act was drafted as a result of a Royal Commission appointed to examine and make recommendations on the issue and was the first Act to regulate animal experimentation in Britain. It was to remain on the statute books for over a hundred years. Although in the intervening time the issue of animal experimentation was considered by various commissions, and changes were recommended, the law was to remain unaltered until the introduction of the Animals (Scientific Procedures) Act in 1986.

Throughout the twentieth century then, as a result of the pioneering scientific work of Darwin, human understanding of the biological world continued in a way that would have be unrecognisable to him. In 1909 WL Johannsen wrote of genes (an abbreviation of 'pangene') as the units of inheritance that control the passing of an hereditary characteristic from parent to offspring. This handing on of characteristics is done by controlling the structures of proteins or other genetic material. In the latter half of the same century the discovery that genes are identified with lengths of DNA or RNA was made. As a result, we now know that humans share approximately 98.4 per cent of their genes with chimpanzees. Such information has potentially enormous consequences for humankind. In pre-Darwinian times a crucial distance could be maintained between humans and other animals. However, with the knowledge that genetically we are so close to other species, our attitudes towards and treatment of these species cannot easily remain unquestioned. Indeed, Richard Dawkins, Professor of the Public Understanding of Science at Oxford, has speculated that if in some remote jungle we discovered a species which was a living link between humans and chimpanzees, 'our precious norms and ethics could come crashing about our ears'.

THE VETERINARY NURSING BADGE (Fig. 7.1)

As a final note to our discussion on religion and veterinary nursing, a word should be made about the religious imagery which is used by the veterinary nursing profession. In the United Kingdom, the first Animal Nursing Auxiliaries qualified in 1963 and their names and qualifications were recognised by the Royal College of Veterinary Surgeons. In adopting a metal and enamel brooch-like badge, similar to those worn by nurses in human hospitals, these nursing auxiliaries chose the image of St Francis of Assisi to be the dominant emblem. When their professional name was changed to that of Veterinary Nurse, the same image was used and the Royal College of Veterinary Surgeons approved this use (or at least did not demur from it) from the start. In 1965 when the British Animal Nursing Auxiliary Association was founded (the forerunner of the present day British Veterinary Nursing Association) it also chose to continue to use St Francis as part of its logo. The veterinary nurses' badge used today, which is a red oval shape with a central

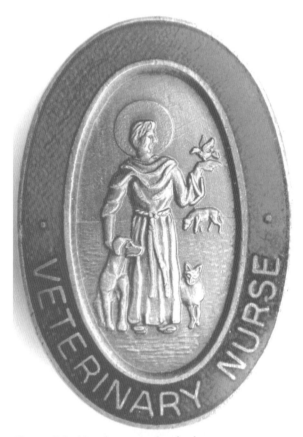

Figure 7.1 Veterinary nursing badge

image, is very similar to the BVNA logo, both depicting St Francis with a cat, dog, bird and horse close by.

The use of such imagery of St Francis seems appropriate. Francis was born the son of a rich cloth merchant but, aged twenty, gave up physical comfort to live a life of material simplicity and to work in the service of the poor (the work of the Orders of monks and nuns following the teaching of St Francis continues today). There are countless stories of Francis undertaking extraordinary acts of charity, such as exchanging his clothes with a beggar, or ministering to lepers, whom others regarded as untouchable. His first biographer, St Bonaventure (c1217–1274), wrote 'The Life of St Francis' in which stories of Francis's gentleness towards animals are especially noticeable. Francis was motivated in his kindness towards animals in that he saw all of the world as part of God's creation and that no part of it should be neglected or abused (he used to call other created things by familial names 'Brother Moon, Sister Sun', for example). Francis himself wrote that 'If you have people who will exclude any of God's creatures from the shelter of compassion and pity, you will have people who deal likewise with their fellow humans'. Francis is recognised by the Roman Catholic Church, and others too, as the Patron Saint of animals. His Feast Day, the day in which he is particularly remembered by the Church, is 4 October, which by co-incidence is the same month that the BVNA has its annual Congress. There are today countless animal charities and other organisations which use Francis's name. These include animal rescue societies, animal shelters and animal sanctuaries.

Even in a culture such as the UK where there is a multiplicity of religious provision, it can be seen that the life and example of St Francis can inspire both those of religious faith and those of none to a life of service. Looked at in such a way, it is right that the veterinary nursing badge carries Francis's image. Indeed, to catch a glimpse of the badge on the uniform may serve not only as a reminder to veterinary nurses of the kind of devotion to animals to which they have committed themselves, but also to animal owners and others who may be reassured that the animals in the nurses' care are cared for in such a light.

CONCLUSION

In this chapter we have seen that the history of human treatment of animals, motivated by religious conviction, has been both long and varied. Whilst vestiges of Aristotelianism still linger today, there are also however real signs of encouragement from those of the various religious faiths (and from those of no particular religious affiliation) who urge that humans should both moderate their use of animals and where possible remove the need of animals to be used at all, using them only when necessary. While some abuses of animals have been motivated by religious belief (and as we have noted, what constitutes abuse, whether motivated by religious convic-

tion or not, begs the question), it can be reasonably argued that religion today is generally a force for good in animal welfare terms, rather than a force for ill. As the ethical cases below demonstrate, religion can both moderate human excess in regard to animals and also remove the human use of animals in a particular sphere entirely.

Scenarios

The brief scenarios below are each given a heading according to the religion principally involved. However, these divisions are made for simplicity in the text rather than simplicity of ethical practice. As in much relating to ethics, things are often about shades of grey rather than issues of black or white. Similarly, the best action to take might not be framed in terms of right or wrong but might be about two conflicting goods. Thus, where the heading *Hindu*, for example, is given this might mean that the issue involves Hindu religious teaching, the Hindu veterinary nurse, other Hindu participants or might mean that it is of significance to the Hindu part of our community since a cow is involved. The dilemma highlighted might also be applicable, in similar ways to another religious heading. It will be noted that the scenarios are not only about the role of the animal in the dilemma but also involve religion and ethics in relation to other humans. The scenarios are listed alphabetically, by religion.

Christian

Brought up within a Christian household, you believe in the importance of the human stewardship of the created order and of honesty. Polly Miller comes to your surgery for the first time with her cat, Tiger, who is showing all the signs of being in season. She tells you that Dr Quick, a neighbouring vet, spayed Tiger two months ago. She asks the vet to examine Tiger and advise her on what to do. The vet believes that when Tiger was spayed, a small piece of ovary must have been left inside, and asks you to contact the previous practice. Further surgery is obviously needed.

- You speak to Quick and he says 'Oh dear! Looks like I messed up on another one'. What do you tell Polly Miller now?
- What are your duties towards this client? Are the professional and legal duties the same as the moral ones?
- What are your duties towards the other veterinary surgeon?
- What is in the welfare interests of this cat?
- Do you tell the client that Dr Quick is responsible and that he was treating the manner in a light-hearted way? Is withholding this truth in the same moral sphere as not telling her?
- What does your Christian duty to care for God's creatures tell you about this case, if anything?

Hindu

The Hindu prohibition on eating meat stems from a belief in the avoidance of unnecessary killing. It is common in most veterinary practices for euthanasia of healthy animals to be carried out with some frequency. A Hindu veterinary nurse, who has recently joined your practice, refuses to take part in such procedures. This means that she often has time to read the newspapers during the day while the rest of the team get little time for a break, since you are doing your own work as well as covering for her non-participation.

- Do you think it right that nurses, or others, can pick and choose the procedures they are involved in?
- Other nurses in the practice have appointed you their spokesperson for airing their grievances on this issue. Who do you talk to first about this, the nurse, the veterinary practice owner or someone else?
- The view of the veterinary nurse who is a Hindu has got you thinking and you are becoming increasingly unhappy about your own involvement in putting down healthy animals. You now wish to stop assisting with this procedure. Do you think that your boss will give the same weight to your new views, given that you are not a religious believer?

Islam

As part of your veterinary nurse continuing professional development, you are working on a research project concerning Halal killing. You know that the UK government has rejected the Farm Animal Welfare Council's advice that religious slaughter should be outlawed on welfare grounds. At one licensed Halal abattoir, you note that the person killing the animals is stunning them before cutting their throats. Though this practice is not illegal (indeed it is normal for non-religious slaughter) it does render the Halal certification of the abattoir worthless. If customers knew of this practice they would not regard the meat as acceptable. Should you report what you have found?

- Who should you report this to?
- Should researchers be involved in influencing what they observe in their research?
- How far should your own beliefs about the cruelty, or otherwise, of religious slaughter influence your decisions?
- Do you think being a Muslim, or a non-Muslim researcher should inform your thinking?
- Do the implications, financial and otherwise, for the abattoir owner impact on you at all?

Jewish

The religious law of Orthodox Judaism (thus not all Judaism) prohibits sterilisation of animals. As a veterinary nurse working in a Jewish area of a major city a number of your practice's clients are Orthodox Jews. Your Jewish boss is not Orthodox and he is worried about what happens to the large number of cats which are frequently being born to Jewish owners of female cats. He says that he has evidence that most of the newborn cats are killed at birth by the owners. He has started to sterilise a number of these female cats when they come in for other surgery. He asks you to assist in an imminent operation. Do you agree to participate in the operation?

- Does thinking 'I was only obeying orders' justify your participation in this?
- Where is your primary loyalty here? Is it to the client, to your boss, to others in the practice, to

the veterinary nursing profession, or to another organisation?

■ What are the welfare considerations for the unborn animals?

■ What are the welfare considerations for the female cat?

■ Does your boss know of your own religious beliefs? Suppose he knew that you were an Orthodox Jew, do you think he might have acted differently?

References

1. Rachels J. Created from animals – the moral implications of Darwinism. Oxford, Oxford University Press, 1991:130.

2. Rachels J. Created from animals – the moral implications of Darwinism. Oxford, Oxford University Press, 1991:1.

Further reading

Chapple CK. Non-violence to animals, earth and self in Asian traditions. Albany: State University of New York Press; 1993.

A study of the doctrine of ahimsa (not harming a living thing), focusing especially on this in relation to animals.

Legood G. Veterinary ethics: an introduction. London: Cassell; 2000.

Considers the historical and philosophical approaches to veterinary ethics, as well as the dilemmas which might be encountered in practice and research by, mainly, veterinary surgeons.

Linzey A, Cohn-Sherbok D. After Noah: animals and the liberation of theology. London: Mowbray; 1997.

A comprehensive study of Jewish and Christian teaching about animals, arguing that the way we treat animals is a benchmark for the kind of society we are.

Palmer M, Nash A, Hattingh I. Faith and nature: our relationship with the natural world explored through sacred literature. London: Century; 1987.

A collection of scriptural readings, poems and insights from the major faiths. Based on the Assisi meeting of 1986 where theologians and scientists met to define how we should relate to the natural world.

Regenstein LG. Replenish the earth; a history of organised religion's treatment of animals – including the Bible's message of conservation and kindness to animals. London: SCM; 1991.

The long title says precisely what the book contains.

Sorabji R. Animal minds and human morals: the origins of the Western debate, London: Duckworth; 1993.

A scholarly survey of Greek philosophy relating to the status of animals. Demonstrates how much modern thought owes to ancient thinking.

8

Consent to treatment in veterinary practice

Kirstie Dye

The aim of this chapter is to give the veterinary professional an outline of consent to treatment. Consent to treatment is most commonly associated with human medicine and to demonstrate the relevance of consent to veterinary practice, application within human medicine will be considered, with an overview of the fundamental points of consent law.

The role of the veterinary surgeon and veterinary nurse in consent to treatment will be discussed, with specific reference to respective codes of conduct. The chapter will conclude with suggestions for good practice in recording consent. Throughout the chapter, practice scenarios have been used to illustrate the points made in the discussion.

WHAT IS CONSENT?

Consent to treatment is a concept most generally associated with human medicine. In the sphere of human medicine, consent is required from a competent patient for any intervention a practitioner proposes to make.

The word consent is derived from the Latin term *consentire*, meaning 'agree'. The term consent is defined in law as 'deliberate or implied affirmation: compliance with a course of proposed action'.[1]

HOW IS CONSENT EXPRESSED?

Consent may be expressed in a number of ways; implied, verbal and written and in law, all are equally valid.[2] Implied consent may be described as behaviour or action on the part of the person which indicates their acceptance of the treatment;[3] the classic example in human medicine is the patient opening their mouth as the nurse approaches with a thermometer, signalling that they are willing for the thermometer to be put into their mouth and indicating consent to that act, as well as consent to having their temperature taken. For animals, there is arguably no equivalent to implied consent; however, what of the owner? Does the act of bringing an animal to a practice and seeking veterinary advice indicate any form of consent?

Box 8.1

An owner brings his cat into your practice to be spayed. Before the owner has agreed the cost of treatment or given consent, he leaves to answer his mobile telephone. Forty minutes later the veterinary surgeon is keen to begin the procedure so it is completed before evening surgery.

Do you think the owner's act of bringing his cat into the practice to be spayed implies his consent to his cat undergoing surgery?

In the commercial situation, it would be unwise to view the owner's actions as implied consent to previously discussed treatment. Without discussing the treatment with the owner it is not possible to evaluate the owner's understanding of the proposed treatment, gain their agreement to the cost involved or for the owner to ask further questions. From a safety perspective, it is not known whether the cat has been fasted in readiness for a general anaesthetic and there may be other reasons for the owner to bring the cat to the veterinary surgeon, for example, the cat may have been unwell.

Although written, verbal and implied consent are equally valid in law,[4] written consent is often favoured for evidentiary purposes; although a signature on a consent form does not equate to valid consent, it may indicate that an interaction took place between the professional and the owner after which the owner agreed to sign. The requirements for valid consent must still be met and if they are not, even if the owner has signed the consent form, consent may not be valid.

THE CONCEPT OF CONSENT IN VETERINARY MEDICINE

To develop an understanding of how this essentially human concept can be applied to veterinary medicine, it is necessary to consider how consent law is applied to human patients.

Within human medicine, consent to treatment was first considered in the case of Schloendorff v. Society of New York Hospital,[5] in which Cardozo J gave the seminal expression of consent as 'every human being of adult years and sound mind has a right to determine what shall be done with his own body'.[4] This premise would seem to be easy to apply to the human patient; however, the quote indicates the requirements necessary for valid consent; adult years and sound mind. The adult human patient must have competency, sufficient age and maturity and capacity.[3] It is a basic principle of consent law as applied to the human patient, that no one may consent on the behalf of the adult human patient, regardless of the competence of the patient.[4]

In English law it is important to understand that competence 'depends on the particular transaction in issue'.[6] Competence is not a blanket condition,

one is not either 'competent' or 'incompetent' and, therefore, a human patient may be competent for some decisions whilst at the same time, being incompetent for others.[4] The legal test of competence is outlined in the case of Re C (adult: refusal of medical treatment)[7] and has three steps:

1. Is the person able to take in and retain treatment information?
2. Does the person believe it?
3. Can the person weigh the information and make a decision?

It would seem to be obvious that animals lack competence to make decisions and would at all times fail to meet the test of competence, however, what of the owner? If the owner does not meet the test of competence should they, or are they, able to consent to treatment on the behalf of their animal?

Box 8.2   Requirements for valid consent

- Competence.
- Sufficient age and maturity.
- Capacity.

Box 8.3

An elderly lady has been bringing her very elderly cat to a veterinary practice for many years; the cat has a chronic condition which has required regular visits. Over the last couple of years the practice staff have noticed that the lady does not seem to be as 'with it'; sometimes the lady seems to get quite muddled over appointment dates and times and the receptionist always has to write down the details very clearly for the lady and ring to remind the lady the day before the appointment and the day of the appointment. The lady sometimes seems quite muddled when dealing with payment and the receptionist usually has to take the money from the lady's purse and show her what she has taken and the change, leaving a clear receipt in her purse. Over recent weeks the condition of the cat has deteriorated and the veterinary surgeon has now discussed with the lady that the time is right to 'put the cat to sleep'. The nurse on duty is explaining the process of euthanasia and the cost to the lady and requesting her consent and for her to sign the consent form for euthanasia. However, even though, when asked, the lady states 'I do understand, dear' the nurse does not feel confident that the lady does understand that her cat is being euthanased, as she has made reference to needing to buy more cat food and the nurse knows the lady has no other pets.

Would you be satisfied that this lady was able to give consent?

Competence

Children are patients who may often, although not always particularly during adolescence, lack the criteria to consent on their own behalf. What of the human patient who lacks sufficient age and maturity? For the child lacking mental capacity, this is well established in law; a parent or legal guardian retains the right to consent on the behalf of their child.[8] Where a child is judged to have legal capacity, or as this is referred to, *Gillick Competence*, the child may consent on their own behalf, even where this may conflict with their parents wishes.[9] Where parents make a decision which is clearly not in the best interests of their child, the medical team may act in the child's best interests or ask the courts to intervene, as demonstrated by Re A (Minors) (Conjoined Twins: Separation).[10] Cases where parents, who are members of religious faiths which do not support the practice of blood transfusion, have sought to deny consent to blood transfusions for their children.[9]

The necessity principle

For the adult patient lacking competence to consent to treatment on their own behalf, the 'necessity principle' must be invoked.[9] The essence of this principle is that the doctor must take such action as is immediately necessary, in the patient's best interests and accepted practice.[9] Taking action which is accepted practice has its basis in the doctor's requirement to meet the Bolam Test or professional standard.

In the situation where the owner refuses to consent to treatment which is clearly, in the view of the veterinary surgeon, in the animal's best interests, would the necessity principle be applied in the same way? Although there may be veterinary surgeons who would act in the animal's best interests if the owner has not given agreement,

where there is no agreement to fund treatment the veterinary surgeon and practice would arguably need to be willing to fund the cost of the care and in a commercial world, is this viable?

In such a situation, there are a number of legislative parameters and professional responsibilities which a veterinary surgeon would need to work within. The Veterinary Surgeons Act 1966 places a statutory duty on veterinary surgeons with regard to animal welfare and allows a veterinary surgeon to override the wishes of an owner where there are welfare grounds.[11]

Various sections of the Royal College of Veterinary Surgeons Guide to Professional Conduct[12] make reference to the veterinary surgeon's responsibility regarding animal welfare. The first of the 'ten guiding principles' states 'your clients are entitled to expect that you will: – make animal welfare your first consideration in seeking to provide the most appropriate attention for animals committed to your care'.[13] It can therefore be asserted that veterinary surgeons have a responsibility to override a client's refusal to consent where there are welfare considerations, grounded in their membership of the Royal College of Veterinary Surgeons.

Within the section of the RCVS Guide to Professional Conduct entitled 'Your responsibilities to your clients', part 1i states; 'obtain the client's consent to treatment unless delay would adversely affect the animal's welfare (to give informed consent, clients must be aware of risks)'.[12] This section can clearly be interpreted as indicating that where there is a welfare issue, the veterinary surgeon should proceed without the owner's consent.

Box 8.4

Currently, veterinary nurses have to abide by their guide to professional conduct which states that they 'should cooperate fully with veterinary surgeons assisting them in the provision of veterinary care'.[14] It is hoped that this situation will change with the advent of regulation, allowing veterinary nurses to act as advocates for their patients.

Who can consent on the behalf of an animal?

As it may be necessary for a veterinary surgeon to seek consent for interventions, it must be considered who can give consent to treatment of an animal and furthermore, the position of ownership of an animal, particularly a domestic animal. Who owns an animal? This point has been the subject of some debate and here will be confined to domestic, rather than agricultural, animals. With dog licensing it could be asserted that the dog had a licensed 'owner'; however, the registration scheme for dogs ceased under section 38 of the Local Government Act 1988.[15] Brooman and Legge clarify the position as 'domestic animals are property within the definition of the Criminal Damages Act 1971';[16] however, does this equate to the person in possession of the animal being the animal's owner for consent to treatment purposes?

Soave[17] states the common law position as being that a domestic animal constitutes a chattel, a legal term for 'personal property'. In this way an animal can be possessed in the same way that a car or a mobile telephone is possessed; as such, an animal can also be subject to theft. The difficulty which this presents for the veterinary practice is verifying whether an animal in a person's possession is their property.

Box 8.5

A member of the public not known to the practice brings a healthy German Shepherd dog into the veterinary practice. The gentleman describes how the dog has become aggressive and barks a lot, disturbing the neighbours and frightening his children. The gentleman recounts that he has taken the dog to training classes and sought behavioural treatment; however, the dog's behaviour has not improved. The gentleman requests the dog be euthanased to which the veterinary surgeon agrees as, due to the reported aggression of the dog and the previous measures instigated by the gentleman, the veterinary surgeon does not consider rehoming to be an option. The gentleman elects to allow the practice to dispose of the carcass.

Two weeks later a distressed lady comes to the practice to see the veterinary surgeon. The lady says she understands from her neighbour that the veterinary surgeon 'put her German Shepherd dog to sleep after it was hit by a car leaving the body with the veterinary surgeon and that she would like his body back to bury in her garden'. On further discussion, the lady describes how the dog was left in the care of her neighbour whilst she was on holiday. It becomes apparent that the gentlemen who brought the German Shepherd into the practice was not the owner, rather he was the neighbour of the owner, who, on further exploration by the veterinary surgeon, the lady now describes as having been disturbed by the dogs barking, particularly at his children.

Do you think the veterinary surgeon was right to euthanase the dog?

Organisations such as the Kennel Club operate a registration scheme for pedigree animals, which may give some indication of ownership (provided the full pedigree name is divulged), as may microchipping, tattooing and freeze marking. However, how far does the veterinary practice have a responsibility to establish ownership of an animal before allowing the person in possession of the animal to instigate care and consent to treatment?

Brooman and Legge assert that 'if someone without lawful excuse destroys or damages another animal belonging to someone else and they do so intentionally or recklessly, or they threaten to do so, then it will be an offence'.[16] If a veterinary surgeon was to perform euthanasia on an animal as described in the scenario above without attempting to verify ownership, would this be considered reckless? How far does the veterinary surgeon's responsibility extend to verify ownership?

In many situations where a person brings an animal to a veterinary surgeon for treatment it is taken 'in good faith' on the part of the veterinary surgeon that the person has authority to do so. For regular clients or animals known to a practice, staff will be aware of who normally brings the animal to the practice and will therefore know if the person bringing the animal for treatment is not the usual 'owner'. The situation is likely to arise more so for animals and/or members of the public not known to a practice.

Recklessness can be defined in law as; 'being aware of the risk of a particular consequence arising from one's actions but deciding nonetheless to continue with one's actions and take the risk'.[1]

It could therefore be asserted that, if the veterinary surgeon has taken reasonable measures to establish ownership, such as checking for a microchip, being satisfied that the animal is not a pedigree likely to be registered with a body such as the Kennel Club, taking account of the nature of the consultation, the requested action and no suspicion being raised by the interaction of the animal and human and the human's knowledge of the animal, that it would not be reckless for a veterinary surgeon to proceed with a reasonable request on the basis of consent by someone they have no reason to suspect is not the owner. A more pertinent issue in such a situation may be what constitutes a reasonable request and there is some debate around the euthanasia of healthy animals, which it is not intended to discuss here.[18]

Sufficient age and maturity

The second criterion for giving valid consent is that the person has 'sufficient age and maturity'. In the case of children, in situations such as veterinary practice, the issue is not just whether the child 'has sufficient age and maturity' to consent on the behalf of the animal but also, whether they have the ability to pay for the treatment proposed. Clearly, where there is a welfare issue the veterinary surgeon may proceed to treat the animal in the absence of consent, however, this may necessitate the practice bearing the cost of treatment.

Box 8.6

A 13-year-old boy has brought his dog into the practice and reports the dog has been vomiting, off his food and listless for 24 hours. The veterinary surgeon would like to take a blood sample and perform an x-ray of the dog's abdomen at an estimated cost of £120 including the consultation fee. The boy reports that his

parents are at work and that he has brought the dog to the practice during a free period from school. The practice does not have business numbers for the boy's parents and he cannot remember them.

Do you think the veterinary surgeon should continue to give treatment?

In such a situation, even if the competence of the boy was assessed using the test of competence as outlined in Re C[7] and the boy was deemed to be competent, this would not ensure ability to pay. Perhaps more significantly, that the child is assessed as competent to consent to treatment for the animal may not equate to ownership of the animal or the agreement of the parent to the course of action. If there was a welfare issue, treating the animal would be easier to justify to the parent than if not, and it is worth noting that the parent is not liable to meet the costs of treatment agreed to by a child, in the situation where the payment had not been agreed with the parent in advance.[16] There may also be issues relating to the law of contract, in forming a contract with a minor.[19]

The same is true of any situation where a veterinary surgeon gives treatment to an animal without the consent of the owner, for example, an animal found by a member of the public or the police following a road traffic accident. If the owner is subsequently found through an identifying collar or microchip, they may not be obliged to meet the cost of the treatment already administered as there was no consent from them to the treatment or agreement to meet cost.[16]

Refusal of consent

Owners may choose not to give consent to proposed treatment and this may be for a variety of reasons, for example, due to the expected cost of the treatment or the aftercare required. It is a basic premise of the law of consent as applied to human patients that a competent adult patient may refuse life-saving medical treatment.[9] This point is well illustrated by the case of Ms. B v. A Hospital trust (2002).[20] In this case, a tetraplegic patient was placed on a ventilator following respiratory difficulty caused by an intramedullary cervical spine cavernoma. The patient subsequently withdrew consent to the ventilator treatment. The case was heard in court where the point of law was confirmed; as the patient was assessed as mentally competent to give or withhold consent to medical treatment, her decision to withdraw consent must be respected even though that decision would lead to her death. The ventilator was subsequently withdrawn and the patient died.

There is, however, also a wealth of case law to illustrate that in human medicine a parent does not have the same rights toward withholding treatment from their child, on whose behalf they may consent to treatment. This is best illustrated by cases such as Re S[21] in which a parent sought to withhold consent to their child receiving a life-saving blood transfusion for religious reasons. Mason and McCall Smith[9] assert that in such circumstances the best interests of the child will prevail and the wishes of the parent will be overruled.

Adequate information

The third criterion for valid consent is adequate information. In human and veterinary medicine the term 'informed consent' is often used; however, in law the term 'consent' or 'consent to treatment' is used, as 'informed' is an essential component of valid consent and there cannot be valid consent without information.[3] As Mason and McCall Smith[22] summarise; 'to be ethically and legally acceptable, "consent" must always be "informed".' Disputes about consent often centre on whether the consent was based on adequate and correct information and was valid or was based on inadequate or incorrect information and whether this invalidated the consent. Disputes occur less often where there is a complete absence of consent.

The Royal College of Veterinary Surgeons Guide to Professional Conduct states that:

Veterinary Surgeons must endeavour to ensure that what both they and their clients are saying is heard and understood on both sides, and encourage clients to take a full part in any discussions. Explanations should be given whenever possible in non-technical language

and if there is any doubt as to whether the client has understood this should be recorded.[12]

Sidaway v. Board of Governors of Bethlam Royal Hospital and Maudsley Hospital[23] is a significant case with regards to consent in human medicine. Discussing the case, Brazier[8] indicates that any claim by the professional that the other person would not understand the technicalities of the issue is not a valid justification for not informing the other person.

The person giving information must also consider the amount of information necessary to achieve 'informed'. Within human medicine this point has been addressed and again within Sidaway, Lord Bridge stated that there were situations where 'disclosure of a particular risk was so obviously necessary to an informed choice on the part of the patient that no reasonably prudent medical man would fail to make it'.[24]

It is not expected that the veterinary surgeon will educate the owner to the veterinary surgeon's level of knowledge, as this is unrealistic. Again, within the Sidaway[23] judgment, it was asserted that the patient should know 'the nature and purpose' of treatment and that this was sufficient for consent purposes. The owner can never have the knowledge of the veterinary surgeon; however, they should as a minimum be informed of the 'nature and purpose', 'risks and benefits' and relative costs of treatment options proposed.

Box 8.7

A lady has brought her 14-year-old cat Smudge into the practice as he has been losing weight and vomiting for a few weeks. The veterinary surgeon palpates an abdominal lump and x-rays confirm that there is a blockage in the small intestine. The owner is given the option of allowing Smudge to undergo a laparotomy. The veterinary surgeon explains that if the tumour is discrete, there is a chance it may be operable. However, if it has spread to involve other organs, 'it may be better to let Smudge go while he is under the anaesthetic'. As you are explaining the consent form to the lady and asking her to sign, she hands the form back after reading it and states 'I want him to have the operation but not be put to sleep, I want to take him home'. This leads you to conclude that the lady may not understand the full implications of the surgery or Smudge's condition.

Do you think it would be right to proceed?

As the signing of the consent form is often carried out with the veterinary nurse, it is necessary for the veterinary nurse to try to evaluate the client's understanding as well as offer information.[25] If this happens after a consultation with a veterinary surgeon, it may be possible to evaluate a client's understanding of the information they have been given by asking them to explain what they understand the options are and the possible implications of each option. Where a client is unable to give an outline, this may indicate they have either not understood the options and implications or have not been given adequate information on which to make an informed choice. Where there was a welfare issue, it would be possible for the veterinary surgeon to proceed without consent, however, in the scenario outlined above the issue is more whether Smudge has an operation or is given palliative care until consent can be obtained.

An example of good practice which has been adopted in human medicine is that the nurse is present when the doctor is giving information to a patient, whether that be the result of investigations or treatment options.[26] The rationale for this is that the nurse is then aware of what information the patient has received, is able to discuss the information with the patient, the patient is able to ask further questions which they may not have thought of previously and in this way, the nurse may be able to further evaluate the patient's understanding. Often the patient may feel they know the nurse better than the doctor and are more comfortable with them, so may be more willing to ask the nurse questions they did not ask the doctor. The nurse also has more time. During a reasonably short consultation with the doctor, who the patient may perceive to be very busy, the patient may not

feel they can ask lots of questions as this takes up the doctor's time; however, the patient may feel more comfortable taking up the nurse's time. This may be a model of good practice which could offer similar benefits in veterinary practice, particularly as it is often the veterinary nurse with whom the patient signs the consent form, rather than the veterinary surgeon.

THE RELATIONSHIP OF CONSENT TO TREATMENT TO CONTRACT LAW

Earle describes consent as 'evidence of the contract which exists between the veterinary practice and the client'[27] with Soave stating 'the veterinary–client relationship involves the principles of contract and tort law'.[28] Consent to treatment of an animal by the animal's owner could be described as the client entering into a contract with the veterinary surgeon and practice. This differs from the human patient receiving National Health Service care. It is not intended to discuss this highly complex area of law within this text; however, it is of note that the veterinary surgeon is bound by contract law as well as tort law, where a legally binding contract has been formed with a client.

Formation of a contract

The elements essential for the formation of a contract are: offer, acceptance, intention to create legal relations, agreement and consideration.[19] An offer can be defined in law as 'a statement of intent by the offeror to be legally bound by the terms of the offer if it is accepted, and the contract exists once acceptance has taken place'.[29] There is no requirement for the offer or acceptance to be made in writing. For a contract to be binding there must be an 'intention to create legal relations' for both parties and within commercial agreements there is an assumption of intention to create legal relations.[19] The final ingredient for a contract is consideration, defined by Sir Frederick Pollock as 'the price for which the promise is bought'.[30] The person making the promise, who will be the veterinary surgeon, must receive some benefit in return, which will be some form of payment for the service given. This payment does not have to be in the form of money[19] although in the veterinary situation this will be the usual form of consideration.

By introducing the estimated cost of the treatment into the consent process, the veterinary practice is establishing the consideration for the service and as such, is fulfilling the elements necessary for a contract, thus creating a contract between the veterinary practice and client.

Within human medical treatment carried out by the National Health Service, the element of consideration is absent and therefore a legally binding contract is not formed when a patient consents to treatment within the National Health Service. Consideration is absent as the patient is not paying for the service they are receiving. Although it could be argued that payment is through income taxation, this is too remote to be deemed consideration for a specific treatment received from the National Health Service.

The case of Thompson v. Sheffield Fertility Clinic[31] is a good example of how the position changes where consideration is present. In this case, as the patient was paying for 'in vitro' fertilisation privately, the contractual element of consideration was present and the patient was able to raise an action in contract against the practitioner.

For treatment carried out by the National Health Service the patient generally only has the option of raising an action in tort, usually for negligence. The nature of the contract in private veterinary

practice gives the owner not only the option of raising an action in tort if an adverse outcome results, but also in contract.

As treatment carried out by a veterinary surgeon on behalf of a charity involves no payment by the owner, there is no consideration and therefore, as one of the elements necessary to form a contract is absent, there can be no action raised in contract by an owner where a veterinary surgeon has exceeded the scope of the consent given. The owner may still have an action in tort if the procedure was negligently performed or has the option of reporting the veterinary surgeon to the Blue Cross as employers and RCVS as regulators for unprofessional conduct. It is also worth noting that a voluntary contribution made to the charity concerned would not be deemed consideration for the purposes of a contract.

quotes' for the treatment necessary. When the veterinary nurses are asking the owners to sign the consent form an estimate of the treatment cost is given to the client to inform their decision. However, the nurses have noticed that routine costs like antibiotics and dressings are not included in the initial quote and consequently, the cost of the treatment usually tends to be higher than quoted. In some cases the eventual cost of treatment has been double that estimated.

Do you think this has implications for the client's consent?

As has already been stated above, adequate information on which to base a decision is one of the essential elements of valid consent. If the owner's decision whether to give consent to a procedure is based on the cost of the procedure, possibly weighed against the cost of other treatments or euthanasia, if that information is incorrect the consent will not have been based on true information and may therefore be compromised.[22]

The behaviour of the veterinary surgeon, in under-quoting, is also unprofessional and, as honesty and integrity are arguably essential characteristics expected of professionals, this would require action from the regulating body.

THE ROLE OF THE VETERINARY SURGEON IN CONSENT TO TREATMENT

The veterinary surgeon has the primary role in consent to treatment. The role has two strands: gaining consent from the owner of the animal for proposed treatment and taking action where consent is either withheld or the person able to consent is not available.

The RCVS Guide to Professional Conduct states that veterinary surgeons must 'obtain the client's consent to treatment unless delay would adversely affect the animal's welfare (to give informed consent clients must be aware of the risks)'.[12]

Information is a key requirement for valid consent, and although the Guide to Professional Conduct only makes specific reference to risks

involved in proposed treatment, the veterinary surgeon should also discuss the benefits which proposed treatments may afford, to enable the owner to weigh up the risks and benefits of a particular course of action. Part f states that veterinary surgeons must 'ensure that a range of reasonable treatment options are offered and explained, including prognosis and possible side effects'.[12] This section should be read in conjunction with section l 'recognise that the client has freedom of choice'[12] and section 2d 'give due consideration to the client's concerns and wishes where these do not conflict with the patient's welfare'.[12]

The veterinary surgeon should give information in an impartial manner, and in a way which does not lead the client to a course of action favoured by the veterinary surgeon, where other options are available.

The Guide to Professional Conduct continues; 'ensure that the client is made aware of any procedure to be performed by support staff who are not veterinary surgeons',[12] placing a responsibility on the veterinary surgeon, as part of the information-giving element of seeking consent from an owner, to include information about who is to perform the procedure.

It is also necessary for clients to have the opportunity to ask any questions they may have regarding the proposed treatment, which may influence their decision. In veterinary practice, where consultation time may be limited, clients should not be made to feel pressurised into making decisions and should also, where there is no immediate welfare issue, be aware that they may think options over before reaching a decision, as a matter of good practice.

Box 8.11

A veterinary surgeon has a consultation with an owner regarding her elderly pony, Fudge. Fudge has developed arthritis. During the consultation, Fudge's owner has agreed that Fudge should be admitted to the practice for x-rays and injections of a medication to try to control the progress of the disease. The veterinary nurse is now asking Fudge's owner to sign the consent form and is showing Fudge's owner the cost estimate. On the estimate a medication is listed costing £178. Fudge's owner asks the veterinary nurse what the medication is for and the nurse explains that Fudge will now need to have the medication once daily for analgesia and that one box of the medication contains enough sachets for three months. Fudge's owner tells the nurse that she had not realised when she agreed that Fudge should undergo investigations and treatment for arthritis that there would be ongoing costs and that as a pensioner, she is not sure she will be able to afford the ongoing treatment.

Do you think the cost of aftercare should have been discussed during the consent process?

The cost of treatment options and ongoing treatment may be a key factor a client's choice of treatment and as such, the client should be given realistic information about the costs involved in each option as part of the information-giving element of seeking consent. Section 1g of the Guide to Professional Conduct states that a veterinary surgeon has a responsibility to 'give realistic fee estimates based on treatment options'.[12]

THE ROLE OF THE VETERINARY NURSE IN CONSENT TO TREATMENT

Earle describes the role of the veterinary nurse in consent to treatment as to 'support clients during the decision making process'[27] and it is important to recognise that the responsibility for information giving, discussions of cost as part of that process and gaining consent from a client, rests with the veterinary surgeon.

The Guide to Professional Conduct for Veterinary Nurses[14] does not make specific reference to the role of the nurse in consent to treatment. However, Standard 3 states veterinary nurses 'are only permitted to act under the supervision or direction of a veterinary surgeon'[14] and Standard 4 that 'they should be familiar with and work within the RCVS Guide to Professional Conduct.[14]

As the sections within the Guide to Professional Conduct relating to consent to treatment are listed under 'veterinary surgeons; your responsibilities to your clients', it can be inferred that consent to treatment is the responsibility of the veterinary surgeon and not the veterinary nurse.

Although in practice the veterinary nurse may be the person with whom the owner signs the consent form, the owner should have reached the decision to consent to the proposed treatment during the consultation with the veterinary surgeon. Signing the consent form is merely evidence of the decision, rather than the act of giving consent, which may be given verbally within the consultation.

EUTHANASIA WITHOUT CONSENT

There may be situations in practice where it is necessary for a veterinary surgeon to perform euthanasia on an animal without the owner's consent and the Guide to Professional Conduct makes specific reference to this situation. As well as the ethical implications of allowing an animal to suffer, certain legislative provisions allow for euthanasia without the owners consent on welfare grounds, with the Guide to Professional Conduct stating:

> The Protection of Animals Act 1911 (Section 1), The Protection of Animals (Scotland) Act 1912 and The Welfare of Animals (Northern Ireland) Act 1972 provide that failure to destroy an animal to prevent further suffering may amount to cruelty. The duty to destroy falls most heavily on the veterinary surgeon, who has the skill and training to make the correct assessment. In these circumstances he/she acts as an agent of necessity, and should make a full record of all the circumstances supporting the decision in case of subsequent challenge.[12]

Box 8.12

A member of the public brings a cat into the practice. It was found in the road outside her workplace, having been hit by a car. The cat is very badly injured and the veterinary surgeon decides the only humane course of action is euthanasia. The cat is wearing a collar with a telephone number on it. However, when the veterinary surgeon calls the number it is an answer phone. Twenty minutes after leaving a message, the owner has not contacted the practice.

Do you think the veterinary surgeon should euthanase the cat?

son to see when he returned home from school, with the agreement that she would bring the dog back to evening surgery for euthanasia to be performed. Thirty minutes after evening surgery finished, the dog had not been returned to the practice, and the owner was not answering calls to the listed telephone number.

What action do you think the veterinary surgeon should take?

In this situation it would be necessary to perform euthanasia without the owner's consent on animal welfare grounds and this scenario is an example of a clear situation where euthanasia without the owner's consent could be performed.

A more difficult situation is where the owner withholds consent to euthanasia rather than is unaware of the necessity. However, the Acts cited still give the veterinary surgeon authority to perform euthanasia on welfare grounds where an owner withholds consent. The Guide to Professional Conduct goes on to state: 'if the client's consent is in any way limited or qualified or specifically withheld, veterinary surgeons must accept that their own preference for a certain course of action cannot override the client's specific wishes other than on exceptional welfare grounds'.[12]

Box 8.13

An owner brought their elderly dog, which had been diagnosed with severe hip dysplasia six months ago, to the veterinary practice during morning consultations. The dog has been on palliative treatment but has now gone 'off its back legs' and is unable to walk, which suggests the analgesia is no longer working. The veterinary surgeon advises the owner that euthanasia is the only option. The owner states that the dog is her eleven-year-old son's, and that she wants her son to be able to say goodbye to the dog before euthanasia is performed. The veterinary surgeon agrees to let the owner take the dog home for her

It may be that if the owner does not bring an animal to the practice, or removes an animal from the practice where euthanasia is required for welfare reasons, the RSPCA may be informed to investigate the welfare issue and instigate appropriate care for the animal, possibly with the support of the police. The cited Acts of Parliament also give the police the authority to order the euthanasia of certain categories of animals where the condition of the animal indicates this is necessary on welfare grounds.[32] As the authority is contained in an Act of Parliament this is a statutory power.

Supporting clients in the decision for and process of euthanasia is a key role for the veterinary nurse. The decision to euthanase an animal can be very difficult for an owner and the process very hard to go through. Where an owner is finding the decision hard to accept it may be that the support of the veterinary nurse will be valuable in assisting the process and therefore ensuring the welfare of the animal.[25]

GOOD PRACTICE IN RECORDING CONSENT

Gaining owners' consent to treatment of their animals is the responsibility of the veterinary surgeon. This includes the information giving and question answering necessary to enable the owner to make an informed decision. It is good practice to record the information given, outlining the risks and benefits discussed with the owner[12] and this is now standard practice in consent to treatment in human medicine. Information should be given about the different options, including euthanasia if this is an option, along with who is to perform the treatment, any likely future treatment and care involved with each option and the costs.[12] The owner should give verbal consent during the consultation and although, for evidentiary purposes, best practice would be for the owner to sign the consent form during the consultation with the veterinary surgeon, if the owner is to sign the consent form with the veterinary nurse, this should be at a point where they have made a decision with the veterinary surgeon they are happy with.

Best practice is for the veterinary surgeon to give the owner an estimate of cost during the consultation as part of the information giving procedure, the owner needing a realistic estimate in order for their decision to be informed.[12] It is not good practice to give the estimate after the owner has made an initial decision with the veterinary surgeon as the cost of respective treatments may influence their decision and if this information is not part of the initial information giving, it may be that the owner has not reached a decision on the basis of full information.[3] The Guide to Professional Conduct summarises this point well: 'informed consent, which is an essential part of any contract, can only be given by a client who has had the opportunity to consider the options for treatment, and had the significance and risks explained to them. Cost may also be relevant to the client's decision'.[12]

The separation of the consent to treatment of the animal and the contract with the veterinary surgeon or practice is advised.[28] This may be achieved by ensuring that accurate estimates of cost are given as part of the information giving process prior to the client making a decision, having a form recording consent to treatment and a separate written estimate of cost instead of combining the two forms.

References

1. Martin EA. Dictionary of law. Oxford: Oxford University Press; 2003.
2. Montgomery J. Health care law. Oxford: Oxford University Press; 1997.
3. Kennedy I, Grubb A. Medical law. 3rd edn. London: Butterworths; 2000.
4. Kennedy I, Grubb A. Principles of medical law. Oxford: Oxford University Press; 1998.
5. Schloendorff v. Society of New York Hospital 211 NY 125, 105 NE 92 (NY), 1914.
6. Brazier M. Medicine, patients and the law. 3rd edn. London: Penguin; 2003:122.
7. Re C (adult: refusal of medical treatment) [1994] 1 All ER 819.
8. Brazier M. Medicine, patients and the law. 3rd edn. London: Penguin; 2003.
9. Mason JK, McCall Smith RA, Laurie GT. Law and medical ethics. 6th edn. London: Butterworths; 2002.
10. Re A (Minors) (Conjoined Twins: Surgical Separation) [2001] 4 All ER 961.
11. Veterinary Surgeons Act 1966. London: HMSO.
12. RCVS. Guide to Professional Conduct. London: Royal College of Veterinary Surgeons; 2004.
13. RCVS. Ten guiding principles. London: Royal College of Veterinary Surgeons; 2004: 4.
14. RCVS. Guide to Professional Conduct for Veterinary Nurses. London: Royal College of Veterinary Surgeons; 2000.
15. Local Government Act 1988. London: HMSO; Section 38.
16. Brooman S, Legge D. Law relating to animals. London: Cavendish; 1997:227.
17. Soave O. Animals, the law and veterinary medicine. 4th edn. Oxford: Austin and Winfield; 2000.
18. Tannenbaum J. Veterinary ethics. 2nd edn. London: Mosby; 1995.
19. Beatson J. Anson's law of contract. 28th edn. Oxford: Oxford University Press; 2002.
20. Ms. B v. A Hospital Trust [2002] 2 All ER 449.
21. Re S (a minor) (medical treatment) [1993] 1 FLR 376.
22. Mason JK, McCall Smith RA, Laurie GT. Law and medical ethics. 6th edn. London: Butterworths; 2002: 351.
23. Sidaway v. Board of Governors of Bethlam Royal Hospital and Maudsley Hospital [1985] 2 WLR 480.
24. Brazier M. Medicine, patients and the law. 3rd edn. London: Penguin; 2003:104.
25. Jones L, Stewart MF. Managing animal death: helping clients through pet loss. In: Lane DR, Cooper B, eds. Veterinary nursing. 3rd edn. London: Butterworth-Heinemann; 2003:761–766.

26. Dimond B. Legal aspects of nursing, 4th edn. London: Prentice Hall: 2004.

27. Earle E. Legal and ethical aspects of veterinary nursing practice. In: Lane DR, Cooper B, eds. Veterinary nursing. 3rd edn. London: Butterworth-Heinemann: 2003:205–214, 210–211.

28. Soave O. Animals, the law and veterinary medicine. 4th edn. Oxford: Austin and Winfield; 2000:40.

29. Turner C. Unlocking contract law. London: Hodder & Stoughton; 2004:16.

30. Thomas v. Thomas (1842) 2QB 851.

31. Patricia Thompson v. Sheffield Fertility Clinic (2000) LTL 5/2/2001.

32. Brooman S, Legge D. Law relating to animals London: Cavendish; 1997.

9

The Veterinary Surgeons Act 1966

Gordon Hockey

The Veterinary Surgeons Act 1966[1] ('the Act') applies to the UK and describes itself as 'An Act to make . . . provision for the management of the veterinary profession, for the registration of veterinary surgeons and veterinary practitioners, for regulating their professional education and professional conduct and for cancelling or suspending registration in cases of misconduct; and for connected purposes [17 November 1966]'. The Act repealed a number of previous Veterinary Surgeons Acts in whole or in part, most notably the Act of 1881 and (in part) the Act of 1948, and provides threefold statutory regulation of the profession under the general headings of education, registration and conduct. The management of the profession is partly through the Act and partly through Royal Charter that established the Royal College of Veterinary Surgeons in 1844, prior to the first Veterinary Surgeons Act in 1881. The Royal Charter (with supplemental Charters of 1967 and 1981) gives the Royal College of Veterinary Surgeons ('the College') a legal entity distinct from the association of its members, and Bye-Laws under the charter provide the detail of the College's administration. The Bye-Laws also provide opportunities for College recognition of nursing qualifications, which are not provided for in the Act.

Section 1 of the Act provides for the constitution of the Council of the College, with further detail given in Schedule 1 of the Act. Section 1 states that Council shall consist of 24 Council members elected from the membership of the College (6 are elected each year for a four year term), 4 persons appointed by the Privy Council (usually including the Chief Veterinary Officer (CVO) for the Department for the Environment, Food and Rural Affairs ('Defra'), a Member of Parliament and an appoin-

tee associated with the farming industry) and 2 persons appointed by each UK university providing a veterinary course which entitles the holder to registration as a veterinary surgeon (one of whom is usually the Dean of the veterinary school). With six veterinary schools in the UK, there are 40 members of College Council. The Privy Council must approve all rules or regulations under the Act (Section 25) and may, if appropriate, intervene in the running of the College (Section 22).

The headings of education, registration and conduct give the overall structure of the Act and the statutory regulation of veterinary surgeons may provide a reference point for any statutory regulation of veterinary nurses. Paragraph 6 of Schedule 3 deserves separate consideration as the one part of the Act that specifically relates to Listed and student veterinary nurses (as opposed to any member of the general public who may help in a veterinary practice and may or may not be referred to as a veterinary nurse (see page 99)). There is also reference to the current discussions on a new Veterinary Surgeons Act, likely to take shape as an Act to regulate the provision of veterinary services. All views, interpretations or understandings, unless otherwise stated, are the author's own!

The Act gives the veterinary profession considerable privileges to the exclusion of others, and it is these that lay the foundations of the Act. It is these privileges that give the expectation of regulation.

PRACTICE OF VETERINARY SURGERY

Veterinary surgery is described in Section 27 of the Act as meaning '. . . the art and science of veterinary surgery and medicine and, without prejudice to the generality of the foregoing, shall be taken to include (a) the diagnosis of diseases in, and injuries to, animals including tests performed on animals for diagnostic purposes; (b) the giving of advice based upon such diagnosis; (c) the medical or surgical treatment of animals; and (d) the performance of surgical operations on animals'. Section 27 is all embracing and it is this 'whole' that is reserved to veterinary surgeons by Section 19 of the Act.

Section 19 of the Act reserves the practice of veterinary surgery to veterinary surgeons registered with the College, giving veterinary surgeons a near monopoly on the practice of veterinary surgery; a considerable privilege. (All references to veterinary surgeons should be read as for veterinary practitioners as well.) Section 19 also makes it a criminal offence for any non-veterinary surgeon to practise veterinary surgery, or hold himself out as practising or as being prepared to practise veterinary surgery. There is no enforcement authority provided by the Act and Trading Standards or other enforcement authorities usually undertake prosecutions, sometimes with the assistance of the College. The College could undertake prosecutions under the Act, as could any individual. However, prosecutions are costly and if carried out by the College might be perceived as protection of the privilege rather than in the interests of animal welfare, although the latter must surely justify the former. The basis for the near monopoly is presumably that animals should not be subject to medical or surgical intervention, however well intentioned, without proper veterinary justification. Animals, unlike humans, are not able to choose between qualified and unqualified practitioners.

A sense of proportion should be maintained when considering Sections 19 and 27, even if a specific exemption is not provided. It is clearly intended these sections should prohibit lay practitioners who advise or provide treatment to animals, but it cannot have been the Parliament's intention to include every observation and comment on the condition of an animal, which might, if provided by a veterinary surgeon, be considered a diagnosis. My favourite and perhaps extreme example of this is the person who finds a bird flapping on the ground and observes that the bird's wing is broken.

Whether the person is correct, or not, this can hardly be considered a diagnosis under the Act that might result in prosecution.

Section 19 of the Act is subject to a number of exemptions, primarily: regulations by College Council relating to the practice of veterinary surgery by veterinary students (Section 19(3) of the Act) and five main exemptions in Section 19(4)(a) to (e) of the Act.

The Veterinary Surgeons (Practice by Students) Regulations Order of Council 1981 (SI 1981 No. 988) as amended by The Veterinary Surgeons (Practice by Students) (Amendment) Regulations Order of Council 1995 (SI 1995 No. 2397), provides that any student over the age of 18 years, attending a full time veterinary course in the UK or abroad, leading to a veterinary qualification and who has started clinical studies as part of that course, and, any student holding a veterinary qualification granted outside the UK who is attending a full time course at a university or veterinary school or at a practice in the UK for the purpose of taking the College's own examination (see page 95), may (Regulation 4):

a) examine animals;
b) carry out tests upon animals under the direction of a registered veterinary surgeon;
c) administer treatment (other than by way of surgical operations) to animals under the supervision of a registered veterinary surgeon; and
d) perform surgical operations upon animals in accordance with the directions and under the direct and continuous personal supervision of a registered veterinary surgeon.

The College's Guide to Professional Conduct,[2] Part 2, F, Veterinary Students, paragraph 2, provides clarification of the meaning of 'direction', 'supervision', and 'direct and continuous supervision' as follows:

(a) 'direction' means that the veterinary surgeon instructs the student as to the tests to be administered but is not necessarily present,
(b) 'supervision' means that the veterinary surgeon is present on the premises and able to respond to a request for assistance if needed,
(c) 'direct and continuous supervision' means that the veterinary surgeon is present and giving the student his/her undivided attention.

The five main exemptions in Section 19(4)(a) to (e) of the Act are as follows.

Firstly, Section (19)(4)(a), any 'procedures' authorised under the Animals (Scientific Procedures) Act (ASPA) 1986.[3] These are usually experimental procedures and are licensed by the Home Office. This exemption helps to explain the technical ability and experience acquired by laboratory technicians who work in establishments authorised under ASPA. There is, though, no provision in the Act for such technicians to assist in the general practice of veterinary surgery.

Secondly, Section (19)(4)(b), 'anything specified' in Part I of Schedule 3 of the Act and not excluded by Part II of that Schedule. This is the often-quoted Schedule 3, which will be considered later. Consideration of its meaning should include consideration of the text of the schedule, not just interpretation of it by others, including the author!

Thirdly, Section (19)(4)(c), an 'operation' by a medical practitioner, for the purpose of removing an organ or tissue from an animal for use in the treatment of human beings; xenotransplantation.

Fourthly, Section (19)(4)(d), 'any treatment, test or operation' by a doctor registered with the General Medical Council or dentist registered with the General Dental Council, carried out at the request of a registered veterinary surgeon.

Fifthly, Section (19)(4)(e), 'any minor treatment, test or operation' specified in an order made under this section of the Act, provided that there is compliance with any conditions in the order. The orders include those to permit blood sampling (The Veterinary Surgery (Blood Sampling) Order 1983 (SI 1983, No. 6)) with two amendment orders of 1988 (SI 1988 No. 1090) and 1990 (SI 1990, No. 2217), epidural anaesthesia for the purpose of bovine embryo collection (The Veterinary Surgery (Epidural Anaesthesia) Order 1992 (SI 1992, No. 696)) and, most recently, for the artificial insemination of mares (The Veterinary Surgery (Artificial Insemination of Mares) Order 2004 (SI 2004, No. 1504)).

By virtue of Section 28(3) of the Act, the Veterinary Surgery (Exemptions) Order 1962 is also an order under Section 19(4)(e) of the Act, despite having been made under the 1948 Act, some four years before the (1966) Act. The 1962 order provides that 'any treatment by physiotherapy (may be) given to an animal by a ... (non-veterinary surgeon) acting under the direction of a (veterinary surgeon) ... who has examined the animal and has prescribed the treatment of the animal by physiotherapy'. A person providing physiotherapy to animals under this section need not be specifically qualified, but a veterinary surgeon would be expected to have confidence in that person, based on that person's experience or qualification. The College's Guide to Professional Conduct, part 2, F, interprets physiotherapy as including '. . . all kinds of manipulation therapy . . . (including) . . . osteopathy and chiropractic but . . . not, for example, . . . acupuncture or aromatherapy . . .'.

Section 19 is complemented by Section 20, which provides that the title of veterinary surgeon or veterinary practitioner or 'any name, title, addition or description implying' registration with the College as a veterinary surgeon, may be used only by a veterinary surgeon registered with the College.

Under the Act, veterinary nurse is not a restricted title, and therefore is not reserved to those veterinary nurses whose names appear on the List held by the College (see page 100). Within reason, anybody who nurses animals may use the title, even though this does not assist public recognition of Listed (qualified) veterinary nurses. It is understood the title 'Veterinary Nurse' was trade marked by the British Veterinary Nursing Association and that this trademark is now held by the College. This could provide Listed veterinary nurses with an opportunity to pursue exclusive rights to the title. However, until this is pursued, it is suggested the title of Listed Veterinary Nurse should be used to denote qualified veterinary nurses. The title clearly suggests a veterinary nurse's name is on the List held by the College and use by others would be misleading.

The practice of veterinary surgery, as provided by Schedule 3 of the Act, may be a small part of any Listed or student veterinary nurse's practice. The larger part of a Listed veterinary nurse's practice may be the nursing of animals, an activity that may be carried out by anybody in a veterinary practice, subject to a veterinary surgeon's overall responsibility for animals under his or her care.

With the reservation of veterinary surgery to veterinary surgeons (Section 19 of the Act) should there be some reservation of veterinary nursing to Listed veterinary nurses, particularly when provided in veterinary practices? It is possible this could be achieved by College advice that only Listed or student veterinary nurses carry out certain nursing activities, for example, assisting with operations.

The general understanding is that fish are not covered by the Act. This understanding comes partly from the interpretation of animals in the Act (Section 27) which omits mention of fish, unlike the interpretation in the Medicines Act 1968[4] (Section 132) put onto the statute book only two years later. The result is that the medical and surgical treatment of fish may be carried out by non-veterinary surgeons, although the effect of this is reduced by the inclusion of fish in the Medicines Act 1968. Under the Medicines Act 1968 (Sections 55 and 58) prescription-only medicines may only be administered to animals, including fish, under the direction of a veterinary surgeon who has those animals under his or her care. Therefore, any veterinary surgery on fish involving the use of prescription-only medicines must involve a veterinary surgeon.

EDUCATION

Those with appropriate qualifications, who may be registered as veterinary surgeons with the College, include those with qualifications from recognised UK universities, those with (recognised) European qualifications (from the 24 European States including the 10 recent accession countries, 3 European Economic Area States and Switzerland[5]), those with overseas qualifications (Commonwealth or foreign) recognised for full registration or temporary registration, those passing the College's own examinations (for those from the UK or overseas) and Irish qualifications prior to 1988 (Section 21 of the Act). Section 8 of the Act also continues to make provision for a supplementary veterinary register of veterinary practitioners, who practised as of right within certain charitable institutions with the permission of the College. Under this grandfather clause there are ten individuals remaining on the supplementary veterinary register. There is one individual, subject to no work place restriction, still registered as a veterinary practitioner under the Veterinary Surgeons Act 1948.

Section 3 of the Act provides that 'a recognition order' may be made for UK universities providing a course of study and examination leading to a veterinary degree, where 'it appears to the Privy Council, after consultation with the Council of the College, that the courses of study and examination are such as sufficiently to guarantee that holders of the degree will have acquired the knowledge and skill needed for the efficient practice of veterinary surgery'. Section 4 of the Act provides that the College may hold examinations for veterinary students where there is no recognition order in force, and this may become appropriate for a new veterinary school such as Nottingham University's proposed new veterinary school. There are currently six veterinary schools with recognition orders, those at Bristol (SI 1950, No. 1301), Cambridge (SI 1953, No. 404), Edinburgh (SI 1952, No. 1602), Glasgow (SI 1951, No. 571), Liverpool (SI 1950, No. 1110) and London (SI 1952, No. 959). The College is responsible for ensuring these courses are of the appropriate standard (Section 5(1)) and has powers to visit these schools and any other universities that 'provide or propose to provide courses leading to examination by the College ... and report on the course, staffing, accommodation and equipment available for training in veterinary surgery' (Section 5(2) of the Act), and 'the sufficiency of the examinations' or related matters (Section 5(3) of the Act). A university may also be requested to provide the College with information on its veterinary course (Section 5(5) of the Act) and the College requests certain information annually.

The Privy Council must be provided with any report to Council (Section 5 of the Act) and has power (Section 3 of the Act) to revoke or revive any university's recognition order, at the same time varying the composition of College Council as appropriate (Section 1 of the Act). The College visits universities approximately every eight years.

A veterinary nurse's name is included on the List held by the College on completion of the certificate in veterinary nursing. The certificate is awarded with a National Veterinary Qualification Level 3, and the Qualifications and Curriculum Authority accredits the College as the awarding body for the certificate. The List of veterinary nurses held by the College is referred to in paragraph 6 of Schedule 3 to the Act, but there is no provision in the Act for the qualification that leads to inclusion in the List. Consequently, the granting of the certificate in veterinary nursing (and the advanced diplomas in veterinary nursing) by the College is made through Bye-Laws under the Royal Charter: The Veterinary Nursing Bye-Laws 2002 (and the Diplomas in Advanced Veterinary Nursing Bye-Laws 1989, as amended). Appeals against all examinations held by the College are provided for in the Examination Appeals Rules 1999, again made under the authority of the Royal Charter. Appeals may only be made against the 'conduct of the examination' (Rule 5(2)), and 'not the marks awarded or other academic judgement' of the examiners (Rule 5(3)). Some provision for the certificate in veterinary nursing could be made in any future Veterinary Surgeons Act, if provision is also to be made for the registration and regulation of Listed veterinary nurses. To some, these are the hallmarks of professional status.

Free movement of workers is a fundamental principle of European integration and veterinary surgeons and Listed veterinary nurses are free to be recognised and work as such, in any Member State. The free movement of veterinary surgeons is provided for primarily in a sectoral directive, which relates to veterinary surgeons (Community Council Directive No. 78/1026/EEC). This was implemented in Section 5A of the Act (by the Veterinary Surgeons Qualifications (EEC Recognition) Order 1980 (SI 1980, No. 1951) with subsequent amendments), and provides detailed criteria for registration with the College. Broadly, there are three ways in which a veterinary surgeon registered in another Member State may register with the College. The applicant may either hold a veterinary qualification that complies with the training directive (Community Council. Directive No. 78/1027/EEC), hold a qualification that is treated as equivalent by that other Member State, or have practised for three consecutive years in the five years preceding the application. There have been further developments on European registration procedures and, for example, third country qualifications (those from outside Europe) that lead to registration in a Member State must now be taken into account in any application.

As an alternative to full registration with the College, European registered veterinary surgeons may provide services in the UK, by simply notifying the College. The provision of services applies to European registered veterinary surgeons accompanying animals brought to the UK for various events, but it is unclear how long a European veterinary surgeon may provide such services before any requirement to register with the College arises.

Section 6 of the Act provides for the recognition of Commonwealth or foreign veterinary qualifications either for automatic registration, or for examination by the College (known as the statutory membership examination) for those with veterinary qualifications not recognised, and Section 7 provides for temporary registration.

Recognised overseas qualifications are currently those from Australia and New Zealand (latest agreement dated June 2000), the Republic of South Africa (only the BVSc. from the University of Pretoria), the United States of America (following the College's agreement with the American Veterinary Medical Association (AVMA), effective from 1 March 2001, and Canada (prior to 1 March 2001). After this date the qualifications were included in the AVMA agreement). To qualify for registration under the AVMA agreement the degree must have been AVMA accredited at the time it was awarded, the AVMA accreditation report must have been deemed satisfactory by the College and the applicant must also have a satisfactory passing score in the North American Veterinary Licensing Examinations. Furthermore, the applicant must not have previously failed an attempt at the College's statutory membership examination.

The College's statutory membership examination is for those with appropriate overseas veterinary qualifications not otherwise recognised by the College and is held annually. Such candidates are often employed by practices as students in preparation for the examination.

The College grants temporary registration for a period of postgraduate study, generally for five years. Exceptionally the College may grant temporary registration for employment in practice and may exceptionally grant a second five year period of temporary registration. Generally, the College grants temporary registration for those not covered by automatic agreements.

REGISTRATION

The register of veterinary surgeons held by the College is a public register which must include the 'name, address and qualification' of each veterinary surgeon whose name is included. According to the Act, the register is to be divided into four parts: the first general list to include those with UK recognised qualifications, those who have studied in the UK and passed an examination set by the College and those with European recognised qualifications or registrations; the second list to include those who hold a Commonwealth qualification; the third list to include those with a foreign qualification and the fourth list to include those on the temporary register. This information is provided in the register, but it is set out as lists of practising (home and overseas) and non-practising members, followed by the lists for the Republic of Ireland practising members, those on the temporary list, and the few remaining on the supplementary veterinary register. The College's day to day working register is held electronically.

Sections 9 to 14 of the Act give the basic framework for maintaining the register and provide that a registrar shall maintain the register and carry out any other duties at the direction of the College's Council. The registrar is the chief executive of the College, managing the administration of the College primarily though Council and its Committees, which make policy decisions and managing the employees of the College who give effect to those policy decisions. The registrar also ensures that the College fulfils its statutory duties. The detail of the registration rules and the annual fees are provided for under statutory instrument made under Section 11 of the Act. Every fee increase must be approved by the Privy Council.

The registration rules changed significantly in 2003 with the Veterinary Surgeons and Veterinary Practitioners (Registration) Regulations Order of Council 2003 (SI 2003 No. 3342), which brought in the distinction between practising and non-practising members, with different fees payable accordingly. Whether a veterinary surgeon is deemed to be practising or not is primarily based on whether activities reserved to veterinary surgeons under the Act are carried out by that veterinary surgeon. However, this narrow starting point is considerably widened by Regulation 24, the use of which has meant that generally veterinary surgeons are deemed to be in practice if working within the veterinary arena, even if they do not practise veterinary surgery as interpreted in Section 27 of the Act.

CONDUCT

Conduct is regulated through two statutory committees, the preliminary investigation (PI) committee and the disciplinary committee (Section 15 of the Act). The constitution of both committees is detailed in Schedule 2 of the Act. This provides that the PI committee consist of the President and two Vice Presidents of the College (who with the registrar and treasurer make up the College's 'officer team') and three other College Council members who are veterinary surgeons elected onto Council; the quorum is three, one of whom must be the President or one of the Vice Presidents. It also provides that the disciplinary committee consist of 12 Council members, as specified in the schedule, with a quorum of five.

Lay input, as well as veterinary and legal input to these committees is seen as essential today, as three Lay Observers have sat with the PI committee since September 1999, providing an annual report to College Council. Lay input to the disciplinary committee is provided by College Council members who are not veterinary surgeons, such as Mr Brian Jennings, a Privy Council nominee on Council and the current Chairman of the Disciplinary Committee.

The PI committee is 'charged with the duty of conducting a preliminary investigation into every disciplinary case (that is to say, a case in which it is alleged that a person is liable to have his name removed from the register or to have his registration suspended . . .) and deciding whether the case should be referred to the disciplinary committee' (Section 15(1) of the Act). Decisions of the PI committee are subject to judicial review in the High Court, although such review is not on the merits of the case, but generally on the College's procedures that arrive at the decision. Recent case law involving the equivalent committee at the General Medical Council (the regulatory authority for medical practitioners) has indicated that the PI committee should not make substantial evidential decisions on disputed facts, and that a complaint against a veterinary surgeon should proceed to an inquiry by the disciplinary committee unless the PI committee can explain why this should not take place (Toth v. GMC[6] and Richards v. GMC[7]). Whether sufficient reasons have been given may also be subject to judicial review. The College's annual report for 2001 states that 'the emphasis of the complaints procedure has also been confirmed as follows: rather than justifying any referral to the PI committee/Disciplinary committee, any decision *not* to refer a complaint to . . . (these committees) . . . must be justified. The difference is subtle but profound'. This change and the higher profile of professional self-regulation, has probably accounted for increasing costs of such regulation for the College.[8]

The PI committee does not consider every complaint against a veterinary surgeon, with complaints handling or screening procedures in place in advance of the committee. These procedures are set out in Part 2, I of the College's Guide to Professional Conduct and initially aim to identify the issues in any complaint. Identification of the issues helps to focus attention on what the College can address and manages complainants' expectations. For example, under the Act there is no provision to compensate a complainant, award a refund, or reduce a bill, and no provision to adjudicate on allegations of negligence, all of which may be a source of discontent.

The Veterinary Surgeons and Veterinary Practitioners (Disciplinary Committee) (Procedure and Evidence) Rules Order of Council 2004 (SI 2004, No. 1680), made under Schedule 2 of the Act, sets out the procedures of the disciplinary committee, while Section 16 of the Act provides the sanctions that may be imposed on a veterinary surgeon following an inquiry. If a veterinary surgeon is found guilty of 'disgraceful conduct in a professional respect' (Section 16(1)(b) of the Act), in relation to a conduct charge, or 'unfit to practise' (Section 16(1)(a) of the Act) in relation to a conviction (neither of which need include moral turpitude and therefore include the happy incompetent), sanctions can be imposed. The possible sanctions are a direction that the veterinary surgeon's name be removed (struck off) or suspended from the register (Section 16 of the Act and Rule 18.4) or a reprimand or warning as to future conduct (Rule 18.4). Although the latter two are not provided for by the Act, the greater, a strike off or suspension, is generally accepted to include the lesser, a reprimand or warning, and therefore permitted in the rules. A direction to strike off or suspend a member is subject to a 28-day appeal period during which time an appeal may be lodged with the Privy Council (Section 17 of the Act). If an appeal is lodged, any direction by the disciplinary committee does not come into effect until the appeal is withdrawn or dismissed (lost). If the appeal is successful, the direction is quashed and the case may be remitted back to the disciplinary committee for further consideration (for example, the inquiry into Mr M Jones in January 2001[9], following his appeal to the Privy Council[10]) or dismissed (Mr Plenderleith's appeal to the Privy Council[11]).

In cases where a name is struck off the register or suspended, the individual may apply for restoration 10 months after the date of removal or suspension (Section 18 of the Act). The detail of the procedure is provided in the disciplinary committee rules and a key rule is 20.5 which provides that prior to the hearing the 'Chairman (of the disciplinary committee) or the solicitor (presenting the facts of the case for the College) may invite the applicant to provide any further evidence, including evidence concerning the applicant's identity, character and conduct since his name was removed from the Register'. Under this provision the applicant may be notified of relevant issues that are likely to be of interest to the disciplinary committee considering the application for restoration.

The European Convention on Human Rights is set out in a Schedule to the Human Rights Act 1998[12] and provides in Article 6 that in relevant circumstances, a person is entitled to a 'fair and public hearing within a reasonable time by an independent and impartial tribunal'. For the College, one relevant issue in relation to this is public perception of the disciplinary committee. Half the members of the PI Committee are officers of Council, members of the executive, and the PI committee refers cases to a disciplinary committee that consists of other Council members under the leadership of that executive. In addition, the Council as a whole approves the College's Guide to Professional Conduct, breach of which can result in referral to the disciplinary committee. The perception could be that Council members on the disciplinary committee will simply follow the lead of members of the executive who have referred a case, or will not be sufficiently independent to act as arbiters of misconduct and simply follow the College's Guide to Professional Conduct as an unassailable, self-approved rule book.

Any human rights defects in the College's disciplinary system are rectified by the appeal to the Privy Council, which provides a full re-hearing of the inquiry and is clearly an independent and impartial tribunal for the purposes of the Human Rights Act 1998. In addition, the Human Rights Act 1998 Section 6(1)(2)(a) provides that any defect in a system caused by primary legislation, for example an Act of Parliament, shall not result in an action against the authority in question, if the authority could not have acted differently. Since the constitution of the PI and disciplinary committees are set out in the (1966) Act the College is protected by this provision as well. However, public perception of the College's disciplinary committee alone provides good reason for a new Veterinary Surgeons Act.

The disciplinary committee procedures are civil rather than criminal and provide for the management of proceedings prior to a hearing. With the consent of the parties, evidence may be placed before the disciplinary committee (Rule 9.1) and the legal assessor can indicate the advice to be given on legal disputes between the parties (Rule 9.2). The rules also provide for the management of inquiries postponed following a hearing, and in such cases undertakings may be sought from the respondent veterinary surgeon (Rule 18.3) with any given included in the written record of the disciplinary committee's decision. The rules also state that any charge that may result in the removal of a veterinary surgeon's name from the register must be proved to 'the highest civil standard; so

that it is sure' (SI 2004, No. 1680, rule 23.6). This is tantamount to the criminal standard and in effect, the 2004 rules have maintained the long-standing practice of the disciplinary committee to use the criminal standard for disciplinary hearings.

Section 16 of the Act provides that conviction cases only warrant sanction by the disciplinary committee if they render the respondent 'unfit to practise veterinary surgery'. There can be argument that only convictions so serious as to warrant a strike off – where a veterinary surgeon is unfit to practise – are caught under this provision. However, this phrase 'unfit to practise' must be a term of art equivalent to a finding of 'disgraceful conduct in a professional respect', because following a guilty finding on either a conviction or conduct charge, a veterinary surgeon may be only reprimanded or warned as to his future conduct.

There are ongoing discussions in the College on a possible system of regulation for Listed veterinary nurses and any model could be based on the existing complaints and disciplinary procedures for veterinary surgeons. The critical question for the College will be whether mandatory regulation can be imposed on Listed veterinary nurses in the absence of such provisions in the Act. Generally any activities authorised by statute may be removed only as provided by statute. The activities authorised to Listed veterinary nurses by statute are those under paragraph 6 of Schedule 3 of the Act (see page 163) and there is no provision in the Act for removing these activities from Listed veterinary nurses. The problem will need to be resolved, or avoided by a system of voluntary regulation similar to the College's Practice Standards Scheme, for the College to be able to introduce any regulation of Listed veterinary nurses.

Until there is some form of regulation, employers of veterinary nurses are well advised to ask potential employees to obtain confirmation of any (or no) criminal records, because the College has no power to remove names from its List, even where a Listed veterinary nurse is convicted of relevant offences, for example, theft of drugs controlled under the Misuse of Drugs Act 1971.

A Listed veterinary nurse may be asked by a veterinary surgeon to carry out unlawful veterinary surgery, procedures not within paragraph 6 of

Schedule 3 of the Act, and in such cases a Listed veterinary nurse could be prosecuted. However, in the disciplinary inquiry into Mr Lonsdale in 2004[9], the College pursued the veterinary surgeon under whose direction or authority the nurses had acted, and the Listed veterinary nurse who carried out the unlawful acts gave evidence at the inquiry. The Listed veterinary nurse had spayed cats and dogs and removed tumours and adventitious masses from at least one animal, practising veterinary surgery beyond the scope of paragraph 6 of Schedule 3 of the Act. Mr Lonsdale's name was struck off the register at the direction of the disciplinary committee.

Developments in professional regulation in the last ten years or so include provision for consideration of health matters, where the underlying problem is considered to be due to a medical condition, and consideration of (clinical) performance issues that generally are not sufficiently serious to amount to removal from the register. Any system designed for Listed veterinary nurses would probably seek to include such developments, but it is questionable whether it would be politically justifiable or financially cost effective for the College to administer such a system before the regulation of veterinary surgeons includes such provisions.

SCHEDULE 3

Schedule 3 of the Act, and paragraph 6 in particular, directly relate to Listed and student veterinary nurses.

Schedule 3 is provided for by Section 19(4)(b) of the Act. Part I of Schedule 3 provides exemptions from the restriction on practice imposed by Section 19, but does not authorise the carrying out of anything specified in Part II. Part II, for example includes '(a) the castration of a male animal being (i) a horse, pony, ass or mule, (ii) a bull, boar or goat which has reached the age of two months, (iii) a ram which has reached the age of three months, or (iv) a cat or dog', and '(b) the spaying of a cat or dog', as well as later in the paragraph, '(i) the dehorning or disbudding of a sheep or goat, except the trimming of the insensitive tip of an ingrowing horn which, if left untreated, could cause pain or distress'. Generally, these activities may be carried out only by a veterinary surgeon.

The Protection of Animals (Anaesthetics) Acts 1954 as amended by the 1964 Act of the same name[13], links into a number of the species and ages set out in Schedule 3 of the Act, stating that if an operation on such an animal over the specified months is carried out without the use of anaesthetic administered to prevent pain during the operation, the operation will have been carried out 'without due care and humanity'. This is an offence under the Protection of Animals Act 1911, the principle Act. (A replacement to this Act is proposed in the recent Animal Welfare Bill[14]).

Part 1 of Schedule 3 authorises an owner or any member of the owner's household or any employee to administer any 'minor medical treatment' (Paragraph 1). Minor medical treatment is generally considered to include administration of medicines by mouth and the subcutaneous route. This exemption authorises the veterinary surgery by which the medicine is administered to the animal. If the medicine is a prescription-only medicine, in addition, an owner, or anybody other than a veterinary surgeon, must administer the medicine under the direction of a veterinary surgeon (Section 58 of the Medicines Act 1968).

Owners of animals used in agriculture (farmers), and those employed or engaged for the care of such animals are permitted to carry out 'any medical treatment or minor surgery, not involving entry into a body cavity' (Paragraph 2), provided that there is no 'reward' for the treatment or operations carried out. Therefore, presumably such persons cannot act as providers of a commercial service to farmers. It is notable that this provision for farmers is similar to that for Listed veterinary nurses, although farmers may carry out the permitted veterinary surgery without veterinary direction.

Anybody, including Listed or student veterinary nurses, may provide 'first aid for the purpose of saving life or relieving pain or suffering' (Paragraph 3), and this may account to some extent for the College's determination at its March 2005 Council meeting to continue to require veterinary surgeons in practice to provide 24-hour emergency cover; thus seeking to ensure that all animals can benefit from veterinary attention in an emergency. The College's Guide to Professional Conduct states 'emergency cover means, at least, immediate first aid and pain relief', a similar interpretation to that in the Act.

Paragraph 4 of Part I of Schedule 3 provides that those of or over the age of 18 years may carry out the 'castration of a male animal or the caponising of an animal, whether by chemical means or otherwise' (Paragraph 4(a)), 'the docking of the tail of a lamb' (Paragraph 4(b)), and 'the amputation of the dew claws of a dog before its eyes are open' (Paragraph 4(d)). Paragraph 4c, which was removed by The Veterinary Surgeons Act 1966 (Schedule 3 Amendment) Order 1991 (SI 1991 No. 1412), used to permit persons over the age of 18 years to carry out 'the docking of the tail of a dog before its eyes are open'. Following its removal from the Act, only veterinary surgeons may lawfully dock puppies' tails and according to College advice only for therapeutic or truly prophylactic reasons. The College's formal guidance on tail docking is included as an annex to the College's Guide to Professional Conduct.

Paragraph 5 of Part 1 provides detailed rules for those of 17 years of age and 'undergoing instruction in husbandry' to carry out the procedures (a) and (b) in Paragraph 4 of Part 1, and in addition, for such persons, and those of or over the age of 18 years, to carry out the disbudding of a calf, provided that the instruction is given by a registered veterinary surgeon, any operation is under the direct personal supervision of an appointed person at an institution providing such instruction and the institution is recognised as provided by the sub-paragraph.

The current Paragraph 6 of Schedule 3 came into effect on 10 June 2002, by virtue of The Veterinary Surgeons Act 1966 (Schedule 3 Amendment) Order 2002 (SI 2002, No. 1479) ('the 2002 order') and states:

6. Any medical treatment or any minor surgery (not involving entry into a body cavity) to any animal by a veterinary nurse if the following conditions are complied with, that is to say –
   (a) the animal is, for the time being, under the care of a registered veterinary surgeon or veterinary practitioner and the medical treatment or minor surgery

is carried out by the veterinary nurse at his direction;
   (b) the registered veterinary surgeon or veterinary practitioner is the employer or is acting on behalf of the employer of the veterinary nurse; and
   (c) the registered veterinary surgeon or veterinary practitioner directing the medical treatment or minor surgery is satisfied that the veterinary nurse is qualified to carry out the treatment or surgery.

In this paragraph and in Paragraph 7 below –

'veterinary nurse' means a nurse whose name is entered in the list of veterinary nurses maintained by the College.

7. Any medical treatment or any minor surgery (not involving entry into a body cavity) to any animal by a student veterinary nurse if the following conditions are complied with, that is to say –
   (a) the animal is, for the time being, under the care of a registered veterinary surgeon or veterinary practitioner and the medical treatment or minor surgery is carried out by the student veterinary nurse at his direction and in the course of the student veterinary nurse's training;
   (b) the treatment or surgery is supervised by a registered veterinary surgeon, veterinary practitioner or veterinary nurse and, in the case of surgery, the supervision is direct, continuous and personal; and
   (c) the registered veterinary surgeon or veterinary practitioner is the employer or is acting on behalf of the employer of the student veterinary nurse.

In this paragraph –

'student veterinary nurse' means a person enrolled under bye-laws made by the Council for the purpose of undergoing training as a veterinary nurse at an approved training and assessment centre or a veterinary practice approved by such a centre;

'approved training and assessment centre' means a centre approved by the Council for the purpose of training and assessing student veterinary nurses.

The College provides advice on these provisions in Part 2, F of its Guide to Professional Conduct, and more detailed guidance headed, 'Veterinary Nurses and the Veterinary Surgeons Act 1966'[15] ('the College's guidance on Schedule 3').

Listed veterinary nurses may only provide the specified veterinary surgery when employed by a veterinary practice and when acting on the instructions of a veterinary surgeon who is acting for the practice. The directing veterinary surgeon must have the animals in question under his or her care and be satisfied the Listed veterinary nurse is qualified to carry out the treatment or surgery. The College guidance on Schedule 3 indicates the College will advise on veterinary nursing qualifications that veterinary surgeons should recognise as qualifying the Listed veterinary nurse to carry out certain treatment or surgery (Paragraph 7), and states the College's certificate in equine veterinary nursing qualifies a nurse to provide such treatment and surgery to any of the equine species (horse, asses and zebras) (Paragraph 8). Prior to the 2002 order, paragraph 6 only permitted Listed veterinary nurses to provide treatment and surgery to companion animals.

The College's guidance on Schedule 3 advises that Listed veterinary nurses should be competent to carry out any Schedule 3 veterinary surgery, and have the experience to deal with the problems which may arise (Paragraph 9). The directing veterinary surgeon is also accountable for such procedures, and is obliged by the College's Guide to Professional Conduct to have professional indemnity insurance (Part 1, E1(i) of the Guide to Professional Conduct).

Arguably, Paragraph 6(c) of Schedule 3 could also be interpreted as allowing Listed veterinary nurses to carry out more and more advanced treatment and surgery, as veterinary nursing advances. However, Paragraph 6 (c) must be limited in extent to 'any medical treatment or any minor surgery (not involving entry into a body cavity)', the introductory phrase of Paragraph 6. In addition, a com-

plicating factor is that anything the College advises may be carried out by Listed veterinary nurses may also be carried out by a farmer not subject to veterinary direction. Arguably Schedule 3 should be amended to provide scope for advances in veterinary nursing.

The extent of the treatment and surgery that may be carried out by Listed veterinary nurses is often an issue. The College's guidance on Schedule 3 provides some examples of treatment that Listed veterinary nurses are trained to carry out, and therefore by implication may carry out under Paragraph 6. These include the administration of medicines by mouth, through to intravenous injection; the administration of fluid therapy; holding and handling of viscera when assisting in operations; collecting samples of blood and the taking (not interpreting) of radiographs. A fuller list may be found in the College's guidance on Schedule 3 (Paragraphs 16 and 17). The list is not exhaustive and nor is the further clarification provided by the College's Disciplinary inquiry into Mr Lonsdale in 2004 (see page 99). By leaving the ambit of Paragraph 6 to individual interpretation, based on general principles, there are advantages to both veterinary surgeons and Listed veterinary nurses, as it is then at least arguable that developments, rather than advances, in veterinary nursing are within its remit.

The College's guidance on Schedule 3 provides specific guidance on anaesthesia (one subparagraph in Paragraph 17 and Paragraphs 18 and 19). It advises that Listed veterinary nurses may, amongst other matters, administer medicines such as sedatives and non-incremental anaesthetic agents on the direction of a veterinary surgeon. This is in accordance with the Medicines Act 1968 (see page 94). There is a current debate in College on whether the monitoring and maintenance of anaesthesia is within the scope of Paragraph 6 of Schedule 3. The College's current advice reflects the current view that the monitoring and maintenance of anaesthesia is neither medical treatment nor minor surgery and thus not subject to consideration under Paragraph 6. In accordance with this view, the advice from the College's Professional Conduct Department is that any appropriately trained person may monitor a patient under anaesthesia, although a Listed veterinary nurse is preferable, and only a veterinary surgeon may maintain anaesthesia, although, again, any appropriately trained person may move dials at the request of that veterinary surgeon. Again, a Listed veterinary nurse is preferable. This interpretation is consistent with the advice in the College's guidance on Schedule 3 (but see page 101).

THE FUTURE OF THE VETERINARY SURGEONS ACT

The future of the Act is under discussion within the College and has been the subject of consultation by the College (in 2003 and 2005) and by Defra (in 2003). The College is considering the regulation of veterinary services, rather than simply the regulation of veterinary surgeons, and arguably the beginnings of this broader regulation are demonstrated by the College's new Practice Standards Scheme, albeit on a voluntary basis. This scheme, which started on 1 January 2005, includes the registration and inspection of veterinary practices, the beginnings of formalised clinical audit and compulsory Continuing Professional Development (CPD). Veterinary surgeons and Listed veterinary nurses working in scheme practices are required to undertake the number of hours of CPD recommended by the College. The registration of practices by the College may become mandatory under a new Act. The College's current intention is for a new Act to provide a structure in which veterinary surgeons, Listed veterinary nurses and other paraprofessionals have sufficient independence to set appropriate standards of education and conduct, with a shared responsibility to enforce those standards[16].

Although the veterinary profession is leading discussion of a new Act, Listed veterinary nurses are involved. This is not surprising. Listed and student veterinary nurses are the most significant group of individuals who assist veterinary surgeons with the provision of veterinary services and should look to strengthen the position of veterinary nursing in any new Act.

References

1. The Veterinary Surgeons Act 1996. London: HMSO.
2. RCVS. Guide to Professional Conduct 2004 as amended by the 2005 guide update. London: Royal Collage of Veterinary Surgeons; 2005.
3. Animals (Scientific Procedures) Act 1986. London: HMSO.
4. Medicines Act 1968. London: HMSO.
5. Royal College of Veterinary Surgeons. Annual reports. Online. Available: http://www.rcvs.org.uk.
6. R v. General Medical Council ex parte Toth, Times Law Report, June 23, 2000.
7. R v. General Medical Council ex parte Richards, Times Law Report December 18, 2000.
8. RCVS. Annual report 2005. Online. Available: http://www .rcvs.org.uk.
9. RCVS. Disciplinary inquiries 2000–2005. Online. Available: http://www.rcvs.org.uk.
10. Mr Meredydd Jones, Privy Council Appeal No. 18 of 2000.
11. Mr Robert William James Plenderleith, Privy Council Appeal No. 13 of 1995.
12. Human Rights Act 1998. London: HMSO.
13. Protection of Animals (Anaesthetics) Acts 1954 and 1946. The principle acts are the Protection of Animals Act 1911 (for England and Wales) and the Protection of Animals (Scotland) Act 1912. London: HMSO.
14. Draft Animal Welfare Bill, July 2004. London: TSO.
15. RCVS. List of veterinary nurses 2005. London: Royal College of Veterinary Surgeons; 2005.
16. RCVS News. page 6. London: Royal College of Veterinary Surgeons; 2005:6. Online. Available: www.rcvs.org.uk.

10
Animal research, ethics and law
Tania Dennison and Matthew Leach

Almost all aspects of the work carried out in veterinary practice have been developed through research in one form or another, for example, from the cleaning products that are used to clean the practice to the drugs that are administered to patients. Understanding the significance of research and the processes and issues involved is becoming increasingly important. Firstly, as veterinary nurses become directly involved in conducting research themselves either through working in a research facility or by being involved in clinical trials within a veterinary practice, they need to understand the processes and issues involved to conduct research effectively. Secondly, as veterinary nurses are often the most accessible point of contact in a practice for clients, they need to understand the issues and processes involved in the development of treatments/medications and what is involved in participating in clinical trials, so that they can inform the clients if and when they have questions.

A relatively large proportion of the research that is conducted depends on the use of animals to some degree. This is particularly true for veterinary and medical research. Although animal-based research shares many of the same processes and ethical, moral and legal issues as human-based research (discussed in Chapter 11), there are also a variety of processes and issues that are particularly unique to it. In this chapter, many different aspects of animal-based research will be discussed. This will include the range of species that is commonly used, the type of research that is carried out, the ethical and legal guidelines that govern it and the moral debate over whether and how it should be carried out.

ANIMAL-BASED RESEARCH

Animal-based research refers to any investigation involving the use of animals or tissues derived from animals. This can encompass a huge variety of scientific research, which can be broadly classified into four categories according to its overall objective.

1. Applied research, which aims to maintain and improve human and animal health and well-being. This includes:
   i. Medical investigations into the cause, treatment and prevention of disease and the development and testing of medical products and devices.
   ii. The production of genetically modified animals and those with harmful mutations, which act as models of normal and/or abnormal human and animal function.

Box 10.1

For example, the identification of the cause of feline leukaemia, which allowed the development of an effective vaccine to control this virus.

Box 10.2

For example, the development of mice suffering from new variant CJD as a model for the disorder in humans.

Box 10.3

For example, the testing of a potentially contaminated food source on laboratory mice.

Box 10.4

For example, the development of a new type of battery hen cage, which provides the hens with more resources, but maintains high productivity.

Box 10.5

For example, studying the behaviour, anatomy and physiology of birds to understand how they fly.

Box 10.6

For example, the testing of a new pesticide to control potato blight, to ensure that it does not have adverse effects on animals and humans.

Box 10.7

For example, a drug company wants to test the effectiveness of a new rabies vaccination in dogs. When carrying out the clinical trial, the vaccine would be administered to dogs and a blood sample taken at a later date to demonstrate an effective antibody response.

    iii. Forensic enquires and the direct diagnosis of disease or poisoning in humans and animals.
    iv. Improving the health, welfare and productivity of production animals, so that they are able to live, breed and grow more effectively.

2. Fundamental research, which aims to increase our knowledge and understanding in a particular field or discipline, where this knowledge has no immediate or practical application. Although this can provide the foundation for later applied studies, the overwhelming motivation to conduct fundamental research is to understand how things work.

3. Teaching and training, which aims to use animals in educational roles, such as classroom pets, rodent dissections, university/college practicals, the gaining of specialist surgical skills for doctors and veterinarians, and those animals killed to provide tissues.

4. Safety testing, which aims to ensure that man, animals and the environment are protected from potentially hazardous materials, by the testing of herbicides, pesticides, food additives, etc.

The majority of these different categories of animal-based research are conducted within designated scientific establishments, such as pharmaceutical companies, contract research laboratories, agrochemical companies, universities and government research facilities. These studies, and the establishments that conduct them, are regulated and licensed by the 1986 Animals (Scientific Procedures) Act. In this chapter, this will be referred to as 'regulated research', as it is deemed to cause unavoidable pain, suffering and distress to the animals involved.

However, in the development of veterinary techniques and treatments, such regulated research only forms the initial stages in which products are tested and their effects verified in target species. Once the pharmacological, physiological and physical properties of the product have been thoroughly understood, including effective dose and possible adverse reactions, the effectiveness of the product in the target species needs to be verified in practice or the 'real world' in that species, so that it can be licensed and marketed to the veterinary industry. This type of animal-based research is referred to as a 'clinical trial' as it is often conducted in a clinical setting (such as a veterinary practice, farm, or zoo) and forms part of routine clinical practice.

Animals are also used in research that is deemed *not* to require legal regulation and licensing, as it is *not* considered to cause unavoidable pain, suffering and distress to any of the animals involved.

Box 10.8

For example, observing the feeding behaviour of wild ponies on Exmoor to identify what they do at different times of the day and what they eat.

However, this non-regulated research is often regulated at a local (individual institution) level by 'in house' welfare and research committees. This type of research most often involves simply taking observations of the animals and collecting non-invasive samples (e.g. faeces, urine, hair, etc.). These studies are often referred to as 'non-regulated research' and can be conducted in a wide variety of places, including universities, veterinary practices, zoos, animal shelters, farms, as well as in the field.

Due to the non-invasive nature of this type of animal-based research, and the lack of legal and ethical guidelines relating to it, no further discussion of it will take place in this chapter.

WHY USE ANIMALS?

The most basic and universal reason for using living animals in research is that to fully understand the complex physiological, biochemical, psychological and physical systems that make up living organisms, we have to study those living organisms in their entirety. After all, the study of isolated parts or processes does not always represent what goes on in the whole body. In the case of research that is conducted to directly benefit animals, use of the same or related species to those who will benefit from the findings is going to be the most effective way of obtaining valid results.

In the case of research that is conducted to benefit humans it is argued that, although there are differences between humans and other animals, the underlying biology that we all share is remarkably similar, that is, the same organs and physiological processes are controlled by the same nerves and hormones and react in the same way to things to which they are exposed (e.g. situations, disease, drugs, etc.). Therefore, the study of animal biology provides a powerful clue to what goes on in the

human body, without having to carry out the same studies in humans, which would be considered as unacceptable by the majority of people.

In research intended to benefit humans, it is considered more acceptable to use animals than fellow humans for two often interrelated reasons.

- Animals are considered by some to have less of an ability to suffer pain, distress and harm than humans, and therefore it is more acceptable to use them.
- Animal life is considered to be of less value than human life. This is based on the assumption that humans have a much higher moral status than that of other animals. This concept is referred to as speciesism and refers to the act of assigning different values or rights to beings on the basis of their biological species, rather than according to the characteristics they possess, such as the ability to suffer.[1]

THE DEBATE OVER THE USE OF ANIMALS IN REGULATED RESEARCH

The justification for the use of animals in research can be considered ultimately to depend on the objective of the research, that is, who and what will the results benefit, humans or animals, and in most cases, whether the animals will suffer as part of the research. The latter point is particularly important for research that benefits humans. The vast majority of animal-based research is underpinned by the ethical principle of utilitarianism, which refers to 'the greatest good for the greatest number while causing the least harm' and involves weighing up the costs and benefits of a particular course of action or situation. This principle forms the basis of the majority of legislation governing the use of animals in regulated research, for example, the Animals (Scientific Procedures) Act 1986, which governs the use of animals in scientific research in the UK, but generally not those used in clinical based studies.

Using this principle, it is easier to justify the use of animals in research that will benefit their own kind, or other animals, as the involvement of a limited number of individual animals enables us to obtain results that will hopefully benefit an entire population. However, the same justification cannot be so easily or clearly applied to research that benefits humans, as the species involved will not be the species that benefits. It is this difficulty, together with the assumptions that form the basis of the speciesist viewpoint, that has led to the use of animals in research being such a keenly discussed, debated and publicised issue. There is a huge variety of arguments for and against the use of animals in research, which will be broadly classified here. However, this is not meant to represent a definitive discussion of all of the arguments, but a simple summary of the main points (for a more definitive discussion, please see the reading list at the end of this chapter).

Pro-research arguments

The major argument put forward for continuing the use of animals in regulated research is that at present, there are insufficient viable alternatives that can completely replace the use of animals. This stems from the view that animals are the best models for humans due to our similarities, and that only the intact systems of whole animals resemble the true complex organisation of humans. Cell and tissue cultures may be useful in uncovering simple, isolated biological facts, but can only ever be an aid to research using whole animals. This position is supported by the legislation governing product safety testing, which still requires animal experiments in the majority of cases.

This practical argument is often intertwined with the judgements that animal life has less value than human life, and that animals have less ability to suffer pain, distress and harm. These concepts can be clearly seen in the widespread application of utilitarianism, where it is argued that the benefits to humans (of the results of an animal experiment) are greater than the costs incurred by the animals (potential pain, suffering and distress) during the research. This argument for the use of animals in research that benefits humans is often the least publicly expressed, but in many ways the most fundamental.

Anti-research arguments

The argument that animals suffer less or have less 'value' has been criticised by proponents of 'equal consideration of interests'. This ethical principle was put forward by Peter Singer in the mid-1970s in his book Animal Liberation, where he stated that in deciding whether a particular use of an animal is right or wrong, we should give equal weight to the interests of the animals involved as we would to our own interests if we were used in the same way.[2] These interests do not have to be the same as humans, but should be regarded as having equal significance. This principle is applied to the higher order of animals, which are deemed to suffer and so can be harmed by our actions. It does not apply to lower order animals, which are deemed unable to suffer and so cannot be harmed by our actions.

The idea that an animal is entitled to have its interests considered equally to ours was taken further by Tom Regan in the early 1980s when he developed the concept of 'animal rights'.[3] This concept states that all conscious animals have an inherent value or built-in worth, arising from an individual's conscious experience of its own life and the importance of that experience to the animal itself. In essence, rights, whether they are human or animal, refer to 'Quality of life', that is, an individual has a right to live free from harm, abuse, and exploitation, and so experience all aspects of life such as pain, pleasure, fear, joy and suffering. If animals are capable of 'experiencing life' like humans then they should be entitled to the same rights as humans. This principle can be extended beyond just living to encompass death, as animals, like humans, have a right to life. As such, euthanasia of experimental animals, no matter how humane the research, is not morally acceptable. This viewpoint abandons speciesism and utilitarianism altogether, claiming that no consequences, however advantageous, could ever justify the routine and systematic violation of these basic rights, as individual animals are not expendable resources. However, the ability of animals to have similar 'experiences' to humans is in itself a controversial subject, often referred to as the consciousness debate. Although animal consciousness is often dismissed through lack of evidence, it can be argued that the absence of evidence should not be mistaken for evidence of absence.

Even those individuals who do not necessarily subscribe to the idea of animals having 'rights', feel that the utilitarian cost–benefit analysis, that is so often used to assess whether research on animals is appropriate, has a number of limitations:

1. It is difficult to adequately assess what another human being is feeling in a given situation, let alone another species, so how can we compare the experiences of humans and animals fairly and assign an appropriate weighting accordingly?
2. It is difficult to adequately compare costs and benefits, which are not in the same currency, e.g. human knowledge versus animal pain.
3. The interests of humans are often given too much weight, and the interests of animals too little weight in the utilitarian scales. An unbiased evaluation of animals' true interests would show that animal experimentation is rarely justified, except when used in the context of veterinary research.
4. It is difficult to achieve a balance between cost and benefit when you consider that pain and suffering are deliberately inflicted on research animals in order to reduce naturally-occurring or self-induced pain and suffering in humans.

Although these animal rights arguments are considered persuasive, they are not the only criticisms levelled at animal-based research. The need for animal-based research is often overstated and so is carried out unnecessarily, as many of the medical advances in the last 200 years have not required animal-based research.

In addition, the use of clinical human research and population studies has led to advances in medicine, such as the discoveries of insulin, the treatment of appendicitis, and the impact that diet, lifestyle and occupations have on the incidence of heart disease, stroke and cancers.

The statement that 'there are insufficient viable alternatives to animal-based research' is increasingly being contended, as viable alternatives using a variety of non-sentient and non-living materials are developed and validated. For example, the protease inhibitors, which are a key part of AIDS triple therapy, were developed very quickly through the use of powerful computers, which analysed the viral enzyme and predicted the types of chemicals that would block its action.

In addition, many cosmetic companies now use the Irritection Ocular Assay System (IOAS) to screen out potential ophthalmic irritants, reducing the need for new chemicals to be tested on the eyes of animals. This system uses the extent to which a reagent solution, composed of proteins, glycoproteins, lipids and low molecular weight components, coagulates to predict a chemical's degree of irritancy.

Finally, there have been an increasing number of examples where the results of animal-based research have been very misleading.

THE HUMANE USE OF ANIMALS IN RESEARCH AND THE 3RS

The use of animals in research seems likely to continue for at least the foreseeable future. Therefore, those who use animals in their research must do so in the most ethical and moral way possible. The humane use of live animals in research is underpinned by the principles of the 3Rs

Box 10.9

For example, the dramatic reductions in mortality rates from many infectious diseases have occurred due to public health measures, such as improved sanitation and diet, rather than vaccines and drugs, which are now used to treat and prevent them.

Box 10.10

For example, many drugs would not have been licensed for use in humans based on the results of animal-based research, such as penicillin in guinea pigs or paracetamol in cats, as they have fatal effects. Probably, the most infamous case of misleading results from animal-based research is that of thalidomide, which was tested in a range of animal species and deemed to be safe. However, when it was used in pregnant women to treat 'morning sickness' it resulted in the birth of more than 8000 babies with limb defects and deformities.

(Replacement, Reduction and Refinement), which were put forward by Russell and Burch, in 1959, in their book entitled The Principles of Humane Experimental Technique.[4] Although these principles were written with reference to animals used in regulated research, they are equally applicable to those used in clinical research.

Replacement refers to any scientific method that can employ non-sentient material, replacing methods that use conscious living vertebrates. These replacements include plants, micro-organisms, developmental stages of vertebrates before they are sentient, in vitro methods involving cell and organ culture, chemical and physical techniques, studies in humans, and computer and mathematical modelling.

Reduction refers to the lowering of the number of animals used to obtain information of a given amount and precision. This can be achieved through careful attention to research strategies, control of both animal and environmental variation, use of appropriate statistical analysis, improved matching of supply and demand, and the reduction of wastage.

Refinement refers to developments leading to a decrease in the incidence and severity of inhumane procedures applied to the animals used, and/or the enhancement of their well-being. This involves direct improvement in humane practice through research into the recognition, measurement and evaluation of animal suffering in all aspects of animal-based research, including experimental techniques, husbandry and care procedures.

These principles have formed the basis for the humane use of experimental animals worldwide, as illustrated by their incorporation into most modern legislation controlling animal experimentation throughout the world, including the UK's Animals (Scientific Procedures) Act 1986, and Directive 86/609/EEC of the European Community.

ANIMALS (SCIENTIFIC PROCEDURES) ACT 1986

In the UK, the use of animals in regulated research is regulated by the Animals (Scientific Procedures)

Act 1986. It regulates 'any experimental or other scientific procedure applied to a protected animal which may have the effect of causing that animal pain, suffering, distress or lasting harm', which are collectively known as 'adverse effects'.

The Act is administered by the Secretary of State at the Home Office, and enforced by the Home Office inspectorate. The Home Office also considers licence applications, gives advice on all aspects of the Act, and produces the codes of practice for the care and use of animals in research, e.g. optimal environmental conditions and minimum cage sizes, etc.

Protected animal

The protected animal refers to non-human living vertebrates and Octopus vulgaris. It extends to fetal, larval and embryonic forms after a specific point in their development depending on their species (Table 10.1).

Under the Act, an animal is regarded as 'living' until the cessation of circulation or destruction of its brain, so animals under terminal anaesthesia are still protected, even though they are not able to feel pain.

Procedures

Any procedure carried out under the Act is referred to as a 'regulated procedure', and encompasses anything that can cause pain, suffering, distress and lasting harm. This can include: disease, injury, physiological and psychological stress, significant discomfort, and disturbance to normal health, whether immediate or in the longer term. The breeding of animals with harmful genetic defects

Table 10.1

Animal	Developmental stage
Mammals, birds and reptiles.	Halfway through gestation or incubation period.
Fish, amphibians and Octopus vulgaris.	When they become capable of independent feeding.

Box 10.11

For example, taking blood or tissue samples for diagnosis or administering established/licensed medicines.

is considered a regulated procedure, for example, breeding mice that develop spontaneous tumours. In addition, the administration of anaesthetic, analgesic or other substances to sedate, restrain or dull the perception of pain in protected species for a scientific purpose is also considered a regulated procedure.

However, it does not apply to procedures that are performed in the course of recognised veterinary, agricultural or animal husbandry practice.

Nor does it cover animal identification procedures that cause no, or momentary pain or distress. Therefore, the Act does not completely safeguard against harm, but simply defines the conditions where harm is permissible, while making the reduction of suffering both an explicit and implicit duty.

Licensing

There are three types of licence required to carry out experiments under the Act.

- The certificate of designation is required by those establishments that conduct regulated research, and those that breed and/or supply protected species to other establishments. Individual rooms have to be registered for their purpose. This ensures that minimum standards of accommodation, husbandry and welfare are maintained according to the codes of practice published by the Home Office. Each designated establishment must have at least three named persons:
  - The Certificate Holder holds the certificate of designation and ultimately carries the responsibility for what occurs in the establishment.
  - The Named Veterinary Surgeon (NVS) must be available to offer advice on the health and welfare of the animals within the establishment.
  - The Named Animal Care and Welfare Officer (NACWO) is responsible for the day-to-day care of the animals within an establishment.
- The Project Licence refers to the specific procedures, species to be used and the place where the whole programme of work is to be carried out. The Project Licence Holder has overall responsibility for all the work conducted, and must:
  - Be able to demonstrate the knowledge and ability to design, conduct and evaluate animal-based experiments.
  - Have considered the use of non-animal alternatives and be aware of the ethical implications of the proposed work.
  - Be able to justify: proposed procedures, types and number of animals to be used and the severity of each procedure and of the project as a whole.
- The Personal Licence is required by anyone wanting to carry out a regulated procedure on a protected animal. Each licence only covers a specific set of procedures on specific species, which forms part of a programme of work authorised by a project licence. A personal licence holder cannot carry out procedures or use animals that are *not* covered by their licence. This ensures that only competent and responsible people carry out procedures on animals.

Suffering

The 'adverse effects' associated with a procedure and the overall project are classified and controlled by the severity banding and humane endpoints. A project severity band is based on the highest severity band of the procedures that it encompasses. There are four severity bands:

- Unclassified: no pain, suffering or distress experienced.
- Mild: mild pain, suffering or distress experienced.
- Moderate: moderate pain, suffering or distress experienced.

■ Substantial: substantial pain, suffering or distress experienced.

Humane endpoints are used to prevent these bands being exceeded. These refer to the predetermined point at which the level of adverse effects exceeds what is considered to be justifiable, and results in the animals being immediately euthanased. Humane endpoints refine the experimental technique in order to reduce the level of overall suffering experienced by the animals.

Euthanasia and Schedule 1

Euthanasia of research animals is governed by Schedule 1 of the Animals (Scientific Procedures) Act 1986, which aims to ensure that euthanasia is humane, that is, painless and non-distressing, and producing unconsciousness and death as quickly as possible. It states the acceptable methods for killing laboratory animals according to species, age and weight. These include:

■ Overdose of anaesthetic (e.g. barbiturates or halothane).
■ Physical methods (e.g. neck dislocation and concussion).
■ Exposure to carbon dioxide.

The methods must be reliable, non-reversible, safe for the operator and compatible with the aims of the experiment. Death must be confirmed before an animal is disposed of or subject to a post mortem. Humane euthanasia is essential as almost all laboratory animals are euthanased on completion of a study, along with those that provide tissues, those that have reached their humane end point, and those that are sick, injured or surplus to requirements.

Schedule 2

Schedule 2 of the Act governs the place from which 'protected' animals are supplied. For almost all species, this has to be a designated breeding establishment, unless specific exemption is granted. The vast majority of research animals (>85%) are listed in Schedule 2, with most being bred within the institution that uses them, or in designated breeding and supplying establishments.

ANIMAL PROCEDURES COMMITTEE AND LOCAL ETHICAL REVIEW COMMITTEE

The Animal Procedures Committee (APC) is a national advisory body that offers advice to the Home Secretary on policy and practice issues relating to the Act. It also investigates and advises upon issues considered to be of concern to the public, animal welfare and scientific communities, for example, the use of wild-caught primates, and the carrying out of substantial procedures in primates. The APC is made up of a wide range of experts, including scientists, lawyers, veterinarians, philosophers, and representatives from animal welfare and animal rights groups.

The Local Ethical Review Committee (LERC) is a local advisory body within each establishment carrying out animal-based research. It provides independent ethical advice on project applications and the standards of animal care and welfare. It promotes the application of the 3 Rs, supports the NACWO and NVS, and advises licensees on animal welfare and ethical issues. It is comprised of the NVS, NACWOs, project licence holders, personal licence holders, a statistician, and lay people who are independent of that establishment.

CLINICAL-BASED TRIALS – RESEARCH USING ANIMALS IN CLINICAL PRACTICE

Unlike 'regulated' research using animals, 'clinical trials' are not covered by specific legislation. The aims of a clinical trial are reinforced and guided by Directive 2001/82/EEC. This states:

> . . . the purpose of clinical trials is to demonstrate or substantiate the effect of the veterinary medicinal product after administration of the recommended dosage, to specify its indications and contra-indications according to species, age, breed and sex, its directions for use, any adverse reactions which it may have and its safety and tolerance under normal conditions of use.

Types of clinical trials

A clinical trial can be broadly classified into two categories according to its overall objective.

Box 10.12

For example, a drug company wants to establish the most effective dose of a new antibiotic used to treat 'puppy acne'. One group of animals is given an antibiotic, licensed for that condition in dogs, for seven days; a second group is given the new antibiotic at a dose of 5 mg/kg bid for seven days; and a third group is given the antibiotic at a dose of 10 mg/kg bid for seven days. The response to treatment and any adverse reactions within each group are recorded.

Box 10.13

For example, a drug company wants to test the palatability and effectiveness of a new NSAID (non-steroidal anti-inflammatory drug) to treat osteoarthritis in dogs. One group of animals is given a licensed NSAID, which has a reputation for being difficult to administer, and another group of animals is given the new, more palatable NSAID. The ease of administration of the tablets, the response of the animals to treatment and any adverse reactions are recorded.

1. Dose confirmation study, which is used to determine the most effective dose of a medicinal product for treatment/prevention of a condition. This may result in a dose which is a compromise between potential side effects and effective treatment.
2. Verification study, which aims to verify the effectiveness and acceptability of a product under conditions of normal use.

Clinical controls
Directive 2001/82/EEC also sets out that:

Unless justified, clinical trials shall be carried out with control animals (controlled clinical trials). The effect obtained should be compared with a placebo or with the absence of treatment and/or with the effect of an authorized medicinal product known to be of therapeutic value.

Box 10.14

For example, a drug company has developed a new type of once daily insulin for cats. All cats involved in the clinical trial would be given insulin, half being given the insulin under study and the other half of the group (control animals) given a licensed insulin product.

Box 10.15

For example, a drug company suspects that the survival of dogs with clinical parvovirus infection can be improved by using interferon. Half of the dogs in the group are given supportive treatment alone, while the other half are given supportive treatment along with interferon.

Therefore clinical trials can be further classified according to the type of control that they employ:

- Positive control, where the test animals are treated using the product under investigation, whilst control animals are treated with an authorised existing medicinal product of comparable therapeutic value. This could be the same product at a different dose or an entirely different product.
- Negative control, where test animals are treated using the product under investigation, whilst control animals are denied treatment either for the duration of the study or entirely.

ANIMAL WELFARE

At all times the welfare of the animals involved in a clinical trial is paramount. Directive 2001/82/EEC states:

The welfare of the trial animals shall be subject to veterinary supervision and shall be fully taken into consideration . . . throughout the conduct of the trial.

Therefore, all clinical trials carried out in general practice should conform to standards of Good

Clinical Practice (GCP). These standards aim to reassure the general public about the integrity of a trial, and ensure that the trial design gives due regard to animal welfare. These written protocols, based on current best judgement, aim to ensure the ethical and scientific quality of data resulting from a clinical trial. They specify that each individual conducting a clinical study should be suitably qualified to carry out their defined task.

OTHER LEGISLATION AND RECOMMENDATIONS

When an animal is brought into the veterinary surgery and examined/treated by a veterinary surgeon/nurse, the animal is deemed to be under the care of the vet, that is, the owner hands over the responsibility for their animal's health to that veterinary surgeon. This is laid down in the Veterinary Surgeons Act 1966. Veterinary nurses can carry out medical treatment or minor surgery, as long as the animal is under the care of a registered veterinary surgeon.[5] If an animal is involved in a clinical trial, the drug company carrying out the trial will probably specify that the animal should not already be receiving any concomitant treatment, nor receive any during the trial. (Would withholding of concomitant treatment pose an adverse risk to the welfare of the animal?) Any cruelty suffered by the animal as a result of this would be in breach of the Protection of Animals Act 1911 (1912 Scotland).

In April 1996, an organisation, VICH (International Cooperation of Technical Requirements for Regulation of Veterinary Medicinal Products) was formed in collaboration between the EU, US and Japan. The governments and pharmaceutical companies in these member countries worked together to specify a set of standard requirements which a new veterinary pharmaceutical product must meet, in order to become licensed within those countries. By specifying these standards, VICH aims to decrease the need for clinical trials where products are already licensed in other member countries. This in turn should decrease the number of animals used in clinical trials. More

information can be found on the organisation's website.[6]

ETHICAL CONSIDERATIONS

Conducting research as part of routine veterinary practice means that pet animals are the test subjects. Although many of the ethical issues discussed with reference to the use of animals in regulated studies also apply to the use of animals in clinical trials, this area is also associated with a range of issues that are unique to this type of animal-based research.

Importance of communication and trust

The success of a clinical trial carried out in general practice will rely heavily upon trust and good routes of communication between the practice staff and the client.

- Before using animals in clinical trials, the informed consent of the owner must be obtained
- If a clinical trial is to produce good quality data, the vet and nurse need to know that they can trust the client to follow specific instructions regarding the administration of medicines to the animal (e.g. correct dosage, time of administration, etc.) and, if necessary, to return to the practice at specified times for follow up consultations, blood tests, etc.
- The owner taking part in the trial needs to know that the practice staff will be honest with them regarding the potential risks and benefits to their animal. They also need to have a specific contact person within the practice, should they have any concerns about the welfare of their pet. If their animal did suffer an adverse reaction, they would need to be confident that someone they trusted would deal with it efficiently and professionally.
- If a good relationship exists between the practice and the pet owner, then the owner can be assured that the welfare of their animal will not be knowingly compromised. If anything did go wrong, the situation would hopefully be resolved

between the practice, the client and the company in charge of the trial.

Issues to consider before involving an animal in a clinical trial

The costs and benefits of the trial need to be assessed in a similar way to the use of animals in regulated research. This again uses the principle of utilitarianism, and if the costs outweigh the benefits then it is very hard to justify the trial on ethical grounds. Unfortunately, there is no magic formula that applies to all clinical trials, so an assessment needs to be made for each trial. An experiment carried out on an animal is only ethical if it can't be replaced by a non-animal experiment. However, as all clinical trials are different, the costs may be weighted differently under different circumstances. Under no circumstances is an experiment ethical if it causes severe and lasting pain to an animal, or is an unacceptable violation of an animal's integrity.

Suffering to be experienced by the animal
This can be in the form of pain, fear, distress, discomfort, etc. How long will any suffering last – is it for a long or short duration? Does the trial involve a one-off injection, a course of tablets, a series of blood samples or a faecal or urine sample? How many animals are to be used in the trial? Is it ethically more acceptable to use fewer animals for a set of stressful procedures than a greater number of animals?

What are the potential benefits of the new drug/product?
What will be the benefit to society in the licensing of the product? Is there already a safe, equivalent product on the market? Is there a need for this new product? Will the novel product improve the treatment of the condition? Is it society (i.e. the target species and their owners) or the drug company who will benefit the most? It is not just new drugs that have to be evaluated in the practice situation. If a company wants to market a new blood pressure monitor for use in cats, the accuracy and ease of use of this new product will have been extensively tested on animals.

Design of the clinical trial
Is the trial designed to minimise discomfort to the animal? Are the procedures to be used to collect data (e.g. blood samples, faecal samples, owner questionnaires) usually carried out in general practice under the regulation of the Veterinary Surgeons Act 1966? For example, if a blood sample is to be taken, is this normally used for the diagnosis of that particular condition? Is the trial likely to succeed, or is it flawed from the outset? Does an animal need to be used in the experiment, or can the objective be achieved by using a replacement? It may be of benefit to conduct a trial in practice, as this will be the situation in which the new product will be used (i.e. the trial is testing owner compliance, or ease of administration of the new product in the clinical setting).

Positive versus negative control trials
When designing a clinical trial the welfare of subject animals is paramount. The use of negative control trials should be carefully considered, as they often involve the withholding of potentially beneficial treatment from the subject. For this reason, a positive control trial is, in most circumstances, more ethical than a negative control.

Information regarding clinical trials

The following are essential to the undertaking of a professional clinical trial using pet animals.

1. Informed consent of the pet owner. This is laid down in directive 2001/82/EEC:
   'Before the commencement of any trial, the informed consent of the owner of the animals to be used in the trial shall be obtained and documented'. Prior to signing the informed consent form, the owner must have been made aware of the reason

---

Box 10.16

For example, if a company wants to validate a drug to improve kidney function in cats with chronic renal failure, they should not deny treatment to the control cats, but instead should treat the control cats with a licensed equivalent drug to the one being tested.

Happy House Veterinary Surgery,

Catminster

Dogshire

DO90 5CA

6th May 2005

A study to monitor weight loss in dogs fed a diet of Skinny Kibbles

You are invited to let your pet take part in a research study. Before you allow your pet to take part it is important for you to understand why the research is being conducted and what it will involve. Please take time to read the following information carefully and discuss it with others if you wish. Please ask if there is anything that is not clear or if you would like more information. Take time to decide whether or not you wish to take part/allow your pet to take part.

This study is being conducted to monitor weight loss in dogs fed Skinny Kibbles over a six week period. It has been designed and sponsored by Svelte Pets Food Manufacturer.

Your dog has been invited to take part in this study as he/she has recently been scored as obese on a weight chart by one of our Veterinary Nurses. A total of 20 dogs in this practice are being recruited into this study. Ten dogs will be fed a calculated amount of Skinny Kibbles over a six week period and ten dogs will be fed a calculated amount of a non-diet dog food. Both foods will be given to you in a box labelled as either Skinny Kibbles 1 or Skinny Kibbles 2. The practice staff will not know which box contains which food.

It is up to you to decide whether or not to allow your pet to take part. If you do decide to allow your pet to take part you will be given this information sheet to keep and be asked to sign a consent form. If you decide to allow your pet to take part you are still free to withdraw your pet at any time and without giving a reason. A decision to withdraw your pet at any time, or a decision not to allow your pet to take part, will not affect the standard of care your pet receives.

Commitment required from you
Your participation in this study will require the following commitment from yourself and your family:

– Only feed Skinny Kibbles 1 or 2 to your dog during the six week study period
– Gradually phase in and phase out Skinny Kibbles into your dog's diet, as directed.
– Only feed the calculated daily amount of Skinny Kibbles to your dog, no other food/treats are to be given.
– Provide ad lib water to your dog
– Exercise your dog as normal and record the amount of exercise given on the sheet provided
– Return to the practice once a week with your dog for a weight check. This should take five to ten minutes, apart from the last visit which will be a thirty minute consultation with a veterinary nurse.

Please inform us if your pet is on any current medication, suffers from any allergies, or suffers from any medical conditions which we may be unaware of.

Figure 10.1 **An example of a client information sheet for clinical trials.**

Possible benefits/adverse reactions of taking part in this study
Your dog may benefit from taking part in this study by losing weight. Obesity in dogs can be related to an increased risk of osteoarthritis, hormonal problems, fatty tumours (lipomas), along with being at an increased risk if given an anaesthetic.
Your dog may not lose weight and some animals can get a mild stomach upset if they have their diet changed. This is most often transitory.

What if something goes wrong?
'If you/your pet is/are harmed by taking part in this research project, there are no special compensation arrangements. If you/your pet is/are harmed due to someone's negligence, then you may have grounds for a legal action but you may have to pay for it. Regardless of this, if you wish to complain, or have any concerns about any aspect of the way you have been approached or treated during the course of this study, the normal complaints mechanisms should be available to you.'

What happens to information collected during this study?
'All information which is collected about you/your pet during the course of the research will be kept strictly confidential. Any information about you/your pet which leaves the practice will have your name and address removed so that you/your pet cannot be recognised from it.' The results of the study will be passed to Svelte Pets Food Manufacturer and collated with other data collected from across the UK. Once the data have been analysed, the analysis will be made available to the general public via Svelte Pets website.

This practice is not receiving any financial incentive for carrying out this work on behalf of Svelte Pets Food Manufacturer. Your pet will be provided with free Skinny Kibbles for the duration of the study.

This study has been reviewed by Catminster Research Ethics Committee

Further Information
Please direct any questions to: A. N. Other VN on (01234) 376481, or in case of emergency please phone the practice on (01234) 462948

Figure 10.1 Continued

for the clinical trial, its aims and hopeful outcomes, why their animal has been chosen to take part in the trial, the risks and potential benefits to their animal and what the participation in the trial involves for them and their animal, that is, how often is medication to be given, is there a possibility their animal will be given a placebo and not the drug under trial, what to do if they or their animal suffer an adverse reaction to the drug, etc. (Fig. 10.1)
2. Written instructions, the basics of which will have already been explained to the owner before the informed consent form is signed, on what to do if there is an adverse reaction, the trial protocol, veterinary practice contact details, etc. (Fig. 11.2)
3. All medication to be used in the trial must be dispensed with a clear, indelible label on the

outside of the packaging: FOR VETERINARY CLINICAL TRIAL USE ONLY along with instructions for use, batch number, ID number if it is a blind trial, etc.
4. Information available to all practice staff on which clients are involved in the trial, in case of an adverse reaction. This information should still be subject to client confidentiality.
5. Methods for recording adverse reactions of both owners and their animals and accessible contact details for the company in charge of the trial.
6. Instructions to all staff on what to do if an animal suffers an adverse reaction.
7. Information on whether the animal suffers from any allergies, medical conditions, or is taking any medication that could interfere with the trial.

CONCLUSION

Veterinary nurses are currently involved in animal-based research in a wide variety of ways, from being animal technicians and theatre nurses in scientific establishments, to being involved in and conducting clinical trials in veterinary practice. Therefore, they need to be aware of the issues and principles that underlie this important and contentious subject, so that their knowledge can inform their own acts, as well as informing members of the public about how and why research may be necessary.

To that end, in this chapter we have attempted to provide not only the basic issues, principles and processes that underlie animal-based research, but also sources of further, more detailed information on the many different aspects of what we have briefly discussed. We hope that our introduction to this contentious and yet important subject will engage those that read this chapter and encourage them to find out more. It is only by being informed that we can really make the most appropriate decisions about the use of animals in research.

References

1. Ryder RD. Animal revolution: changing attitudes toward speciesism. Oxford: Berg; 2000.
2. Singer P. Animal liberation. 2nd edn. New York: Avon; 1990.
3. Regan T. The case for animal rights. Berkeley: University of California Press; 2004.
4. Russell WMS, Burch RL. The principles of humane experimental technique; special edn. London: Universities Federation for Animal Welfare; 1992.
5. Veterinary Surgeons Act 1966, Schedule 3, Part 1, para 6. London: HMSO.
6. VICH (International Cooperation of Technical Requirements for Regulation of Veterinary Medicinal Products). Online: Available: http://vich.eudra.org/default.htm

Further reading

Books

Dolan K. Ethics, animals and science. Oxford: Blackwell Science; 1999.

Regan T. The case for animal rights. Berkeley: University of California Press; 2004.

Rollin BE. The unheeded cry: animal consciousness, animal pain and science. New York: Oxford University Press; 1989.

Russell WMS, Burch R.L. The principles of humane experimental technique. Special edn. London: Universities Federation for Animal Welfare; 1992.

Ryder RD. Animal revolution: changing attitudes toward speciesism. Oxford: Berg; 2000.

Singer P. Animal liberation. 2nd edn. New York: New York Review; 1990.

Smith JA, Boyd KM. Lives in the balance: the ethics of using animals in biomedical research. Oxford: Oxford University Press; 1991.

Animal Revolution: Changing Attitudes Toward Speciesism Legislation

Animals (Scientific Procedures) Act 1986. London: HMSO.

Internet sites

Alternatives to animal experiments:
Fund for the Replacement of Animals in Medical Experiments (FRAME).

Opposing animal-based research:
British Union for the Abolition of Vivisection (BUAV): http://www.buav.org/
National Anti-Vivisection Society (NAVS): http://www.navs.org.uk/
Animal welfare: Royal Society for the Prevention of Cruelty to Animals (RSPCA): http://www.rspca.org.uk/
Universities Federation for Animal Welfare (UFAW): http://www.ufaw.org.uk/

11
Research on people: ethical considerations

Sophie Pullen

The role of a veterinary nurse extends beyond that of caring for animals alone. Much of a veterinary nurse's role involves interaction with the client as well as with the veterinary surgeon, colleagues and other allied professionals. The profession is surrounded by human beings who possess thoughts, feelings, ideas and perceptions. These, if explored, could help to improve the standard of care given to animals, for example:

Box 11.1

An investigation into the reasons why pet owners fail to give tablets to their animals.

This would explore the issues surrounding client compliance. For example:

■ How useful are practical demonstrations and how are they best performed?
■ How relevant is written information: do clients actually read what is given to them?
■ How much information do owners actually retain following a consultation?
■ How effective is oral communication?

They could also improve the support and assistance given to clients, for example:

Box 11.2 The experience of living with a diabetic dog

The information gained from a study such as this may benefit owners with diabetic animals. By gaining an insight into the life of an owner who has a diabetic animal, a veterinary nurse might be

---

able to offer greater support to clients in similar situations.

■ How do they cope?
■ What problems do they encounter?
■ Do they have any useful advice or 'handy tips'?
■ What do they find helpful?

Or, they could assist with the advancement of the profession as a whole, for example:

Box 11.3 A study to determine veterinary nurses' perceptions of the British Veterinary Nursing Association (BVNA)

The BVNA is the representative body for nurses in the United Kingdom. The work they carry out is funded by the subscriptions they receive. Establishing people's views about the association may help the BVNA to understand why not every qualified and student veterinary nurse in the United Kingdom is a member. The BVNA may then be able to address the issues highlighted and increase its membership.

It is for these reasons that research, using people as participants, needs to be carried out within veterinary nursing.

This chapter introduces the concept of research ethics and examines the importance of the ethical review process. In order to discuss these points effectively, reference has been made to the review process within the National Health Service.

THE HISTORY OF RESEARCH ETHICS

There is a constant battle between a researcher, who is keen to advance the body of knowledge within their area of interest and expertise, and the interests and well-being of the research participant.

Box 11.4

For example: imagine a researcher wanting to study the disease process of syphilis, by recruiting black men, from mostly poor areas and backgrounds, with little education. The participants, who thought that their illness was due to 'bad blood', would be given free transport, free lunch, free medical treatment and a free funeral in return for their co-operation. In order to thoroughly study the disease process, the participants would not be informed about their disease, and would be denied useful medication.

The proposal sounds absurd, however, this study actually occurred. It is known as the 'Tuskegee Syphilis Study'. The study started in 1932 and was halted in 1972, by which time up to one third of participants are thought to have needlessly died.[1]

In order to protect the participants of medical research, and to prevent studies such as this one from ever taking place again, international and national guidelines have been established and are continually being reviewed.

Box 11.5

The Nuremberg Code (1947)[2]
This sets out ten fundamental principles for the conduct of medical research, and starts with the statement that 'The voluntary consent of the human subject is absolutely essential'.

The World Medical Association: Declaration of Helsinki (1964)[3]
This is 'a statement of ethical principles to provide guidance to physicians and other participants in medical research involving human subjects'.

The Belmont Report: ethical principles and guidelines for the protection of human research participants (1976)[4]

It is interesting to note that the guidelines mentioned above were introduced after major scandals. For example, the Nuremberg Code was a response to the experiments performed during the war in Nazi concentration camps.

Within the UK it was not until the late 1990s, following complaints made by parents whose premature children had been entered into a study, looking into an alternative sort of ventilator, without their knowledge or consent, that regulations on the conduct of medical research came into being. These recommendations, from the Griffiths inquiry, set up to investigate the allegations, have led to the development of a framework for research governance, and the governance of research ethics committees.[2]

Veterinary nurses can learn from this. Although veterinary nurses will not be undertaking medical research on human participants, this does not mean that the research they carry out should not be subject to ethical review. It is interesting to note that within the National Health Service (NHS), ethical advice, from an appropriate NHS research ethics committee,[5] is required for any research proposal involving, for example:

- Patients and users of the NHS.
- Individuals identified as potential research participants because of their status as relatives or carers of patients and users of the NHS.
- NHS staff – recruited as research participants by virtue of their professional role.

This highlights the fact that the Department of Health recognises that non-medical research has the potential to harm participants and others involved in the research process and therefore should be subject to ethical review.

Veterinary nursing research will be conducted on clients who use the services of the veterinary practice, and who care for their pets, and peers recruited by virtue of their professional role. It is hoped that 'scandals' relating to veterinary nursing research will never happen; however, it is clear that guidelines and protocols need to be established to ensure that the risks of a 'scandal', or any problems associated with veterinary nursing research, are minimised.

THE RESEARCH ETHICS COMMITTEE (REC)

The research ethics committee is the body responsible for ethically reviewing research proposals. A research study undertaken within the NHS requires a favourable ethical opinion from a research ethics committee before it is allowed to commence.[5]

The role of the ethics committee is clearly laid out.[5] A research ethics committee must:

- Provide independent advice to participants, researchers, funders, sponsors, employers, care organisations and professionals on the extent to which proposals for research studies comply with ethical standards.
- Protect the dignity, rights, safety and well-being of all actual or potential research participants.
- Act primarily in the interests of potential research participants and concerned communities, but also take into account the interests, needs and safety of researchers who are trying to undertake research of good quality.
- Take into consideration the principle of justice. This requires that the benefits and burdens of research be distributed fairly among all groups and classes in society.
- Provide independent, competent and timely review of the ethics of proposed studies. They should have independence from political, institutional, profession-related or market influences.
- Have due regard for the requirements of relevant regulatory agencies and of applicable laws.

THE RESEARCH PROCESS

Although it is not within the remit of this chapter to discuss research methodology, in order to effectively review a piece of research or research proposal, it is important to have an understanding of research methods. Research using people can be either quantitative, qualitative or a mixture of both.

Quantitative research

Quantitative analysis is concerned with numerical techniques of organising, describing and interpreting data. Methods such as questionnaires, structured interviews, observations and attitude measurements are used to collect the data and the number of participants needed to validate these studies is high.

Box 11.6 The composition of an NHS research ethics committee[5]

The committee has a maximum of eighteen members with a balanced distribution of age, gender and ethnicity. It should consist of both 'expert' and 'lay' members. Expert members include doctors, nurses, statisticians and pharmacists. Lay members are independent of the NHS. They can be non-medical clinical staff who have not practised for a period of at least five years, but should also include people who have never been involved in health or social care professions and have never carried out research involving humans.

Box 11.7

Currently, there is no requirement for veterinary nursing research, falling outside the scope of the Veterinary Surgeons Act or The Animal (Scientific Procedures) Act (see Chapter 10), to be reviewed by an ethics committee. While universities often have their own review system for veterinary nurse student projects, no guidelines for the review process have been produced, therefore the standards of ethical review may vary.

Box 11.8

For example: The veterinary nursing manpower survey into recruitment, retention, education and training issues relating to veterinary nursing, conducted in 2004, produced the following results relating to continuing professional development (CPD):

> Three-quarters of employers allow paid time off to attend CPD. Two-thirds of employers fully fund CPD. Seven percent of veterinary nurses can only take CPD if it is taken as unpaid leave. Forty one percent of employers who contribute to CPD stipulate content and 63.2 per cent stipulate budget.[6]

Table 11.1 Examples of quantitative research methods

Type	Description
Survey research	Discovers new facts, often used as a starting point for further research studies or to confirm existing knowledge about an area or situation. Example: Veterinary Nursing Manpower Survey 2004
Experimental research	Allows a comparison to be made between a group receiving an intervention and one that is not – the control group. It is used to examine cause and effect. Example: An experiment to determine whether supplying written information increases client compliance.

Qualitative research

Qualitative research enables the researcher to investigate and go beyond surface appearances and is often used when little is known about the area, problem or situation being studied. It takes a person-centred and holistic approach, thus allowing the researcher to develop an understanding of the participant's experience. It is also thought to 'provide fresh and new perspectives on known areas and ideas'.[7]

Qualitative analysis is concerned with 'describing the actions and interactions of research subjects in a certain context, and with interpreting the

Box 11.9

For example: A piece of research conducted to find out how veterinary nurses cope with breaking bad news to clients.

Table 11.2 Examples of qualitative research methods

Type	Description
Ethnography	Concerned with understanding human behaviour in the cultural and social context in which it takes place.[12] Example: Do people's views and opinions of animal welfare differ according to whether they live in a rural or urban environment?
Phenomenology	Explores the meaning of an individual's lived experience by allowing them to describe their own thoughts and feelings. Example: What is it like to live with a diabetic dog?

motivations and understandings that lie behind those actions'.[8]

The researcher uses methods such as unstructured interviews, life histories, participant observation, diaries and narratives to generate the data, and generally uses sample sizes of between 4 and 40 participants.[9]

PROTECTING RESEARCH PARTICIPANTS

In 1994 Beauchamp and Childress outlined four principles, which are now commonly used as a framework for evaluating research, to make sure that the participants of research are protected from harm and risk.[10] These principles are:

- The principle of justice.
- The principle of respect for autonomy.
- The principle of non-maleficence (doing no harm).
- The principle of beneficence (doing good).

The principle of justice

This principle relates to participant's right to privacy and fair treatment.

Right to privacy

It goes without saying that nearly all research conducted on humans intrudes into their private and personal lives. The researcher may require, and the participant may give, information that is very personal to them. In some instances a researcher may also obtain information that goes beyond the remit of the study. It is important that this information is not used in a way that might be harmful to a participant.

Where possible, all information should be anonymised, meaning that not even the researcher can identify individual participants. Where this cannot be guaranteed, the participant should be assured that any information they provide will be confidential, which means that only those involved in the research will have access to the information.

Qualitative researchers face particular problems when writing up the results of the research due to the small sample of participants interviewed and the in-depth nature of the research. This can lead to individuals from a small group being easily identified. It is important that qualitative researchers are aware of this and attempt to address the problem.

Box 11.10

For example, an investigation into the relationship between a client's income and the amount spent on the veterinary care of their animals.

Box 11.11

For example: A study to investigate the thoughts and feelings of members of the RCVS VN Council.
　The researcher may wish to interview five of the eight elected veterinary nurse representatives. Unless the researcher is very careful about the way the study is written up, it may be very easy for

---

those five people to be identified by other members of Council, and as a result the dynamics of the committee may change.

A research ethics committee would examine a proposal to make sure that the researcher had considered these points and made adequate provision to maintain participants' privacy. For example, anonymising questionnaires, storing data on a password protected computer and destroying tape recordings once the data have been transcribed.

All researchers need to be aware of the Data Protection Act 1984[11] when handling and storing data relating to research participants.

Right to fair treatment

Participants have a right to fair treatment before, during and after they participate in a study. According to Pollit and Hungler,[12] fair treatment includes the following:

- The fair and non-discriminatory selection of participants. Selection should be based on the requirements of the research, and not on convenience or gullibility.
- People who decline to take part in the study or who withdraw early should not be treated any differently to those who take part and complete the study.
- A researcher should honour all agreements made between themselves and the participant.
- Participants should have access to research personnel throughout the duration of the research, in order that they may clarify information.
- Participants should be given access to appropriate professional assistance if any physical or psychological damage has occurred as a result of the research process.
- The researcher should be sensitive to the beliefs, habits and lifestyles of the participant.
- The researcher should be courteous and tactful at all times.

A research ethics committee would examine the selection criteria and process. The committee would also examine the consent form (Fig. 11.1) and information sheet (Fig. 11.2) given to participants prior to consent being taken, to make sure

---

Happy House Veterinary Surgery

Catminster

Dogshire

DO90 5CA

Consent Form

The experience of caring for a diabetic dog

Client Identification Number: A1

Name of Researcher: Beatrice Collie

Researchers position: Veterinary nurse

Please initial box

1. I confirm that I have read and understand the information sheet dated 6 May 2005 for the afore mentioned study and have had the opportunity to ask questions   ☐

2. I understand that my participation is voluntary and that I am free to withdraw at any time without giving reason   ☐

3. I agree to take part in the above study   ☐

_____	_____	_____
Name of client	Date	Signature
_____	_____	_____
Name of Person taking consent	Date	Signature
(if different from researcher)		
_____	_____	_____
Researcher	Date	Signature

Copies: 1 for client; 1 for researcher; 1 to be kept with hospital notes (if appropriate)

Figure 11.1 **Consent form.**

Happy House Veterinary Surgery,

Catminster,

Dogshire

DO90 5CA

6th May 2005

Information sheet

The experience of caring for a diabetic dog

You are being invited to take part in a research study. Before you agree to take part it is important for you to understand why the research is being done and what it will involve. Please take time to read the following information carefully, discuss it with others if you wish and decide whether or not you wish to take part. Ask us if there is anything that is not clear or if you would like more information.

What is the purpose of the study?

At present very little is known about what it is like to care for a diabetic dog. The aim of this study is to explore the thoughts and feelings of ten clients who have been caring for a diabetic dog, for at least six months, so as to develop a better understanding of the lived experience.

Why have I been chosen?

You have been chosen because you care for a dog that was diagnosed with Diabetes Mellitus (sugar diabetes) over six months ago.

Do I have to take part?

It is up to you to decide whether or not to take part. If you do decide to take part, you will be given this information sheet to keep, and be asked to sign a consent form. If you decide to take part you are free to withdraw at any time without giving a reason. A decision to withdraw will not affect the standard of care you or your pet receive.

What will happen to me if I take part?

If you decide to take part you will be contacted in order to arrange a convenient time for you to come to the practice. You will be interviewed in the practice meeting room and asked to discuss the experiences you have had caring for your diabetic dog. In order to have an accurate record of what has been talked about, the interview will be taped. It is anticipated that the interview will last no more than two hours. You will be contacted again within 4 weeks of the initial interview to arrange a second meeting. The purpose of this meeting is for you to look at what has been summarised on paper, and to see if you would like to make any changes or clarify any points.

Travel expenses will be paid to you for attending both meetings. You will be required to complete a travel expenses form in order to claim this fee.

What do I have to do?

You do not need to do anything to prepare for the study, although you may like to consider your thoughts and feelings about living with your diabetic dog prior to the interview taking place. The care and treatment you give to your pet will not be affected by this study.

Figure 11.2 **Information sheet.**

What are the possible disadvantages and risks of taking part?

It is possible that talking about your dog's illness may cause you distress, although every effort will be made to prevent the chances of this happening. If this situation does occur, the interview will be terminated, and a senior veterinary nurse with counselling skills will discuss the issues with you.

What are the possible benefits of taking part?

It is hoped that the information gained from this study may help to improve the care and support veterinary nurses offer to clients whose dogs have been diagnosed with diabetes in the future. It is also possible that you may enjoy expressing your views and appreciate the opportunity to discuss your feelings.

What if I am not happy with the research process?

If you wish to complain, or have any concerns about any aspect of the way you have been approached or treated during the course of this study, then you are free to raise these concerns with the practice principal.

Will my taking part in this study be kept confidential?

Although it is not possible to ensure complete confidentiality, every attempt will be made to do so. Your interview will be taped and once the information has been transcribed this tape will be deleted. Information relating to the study will be stored on a password protected computer in the practice and any documentation produced during the course of the study will be kept in a locked drawer on the practice premises. Any information about you which leaves the practice will have your name and address removed, so that you cannot be recognised from it.

What will happen to the results of the research study?

It is hoped that the results of this study will be published in a veterinary nursing journal and may form the basis of a lecture to be given at the annual British Veterinary Nursing Association Congress. If this occurs, you will be contacted and asked if you would like a copy of the article or synopsis of the lecture. Your name and the name of the practice will not appear within the article or be mentioned during the lecture.

If you would like a copy of the results of the study then they will be made available to you.

Who is funding the research?

The research is being partially funded by the British Veterinary Nursing Association, which has offered to provide a digital voice recorder, and to reimburse some of the expenses incurred.

Who has reviewed the study?

The British Veterinary Nursing Association Research Ethics Committee has reviewed this study.

Contact for Further Information

Should you require any further information please do not hesitate to contact me, Beatrice Collie, at the practice on (01234) 987654. If I am unable to take the call, please leave a message on the answer phone and I will contact you as soon as I can.

Thank you for taking the time to read this information sheet.

Figure 11.2 Continued

that it included information relating to, for example, the consequences to the participant of withdrawing from the study, the protocols and procedures in place should something go wrong and the researchers' contact details. Researchers should be invited to meet the REC to discuss their proposal.

The principle of respect for autonomy

This principle is concerned with the fact that participants must give 'free and informed consent' without coercion[13] to taking part in research.

In order that participants can make an informed decision they need to understand what the research involves. One way of making sure that participants are given all the information they require is by issuing them with an information sheet.

The information sheet should be written in a clear, concise way, avoiding jargon where possible. It must be remembered that clients may not be aware of technical terminology. Where this is used, a definition should be given. It should be printed on letterhead paper.

The NHS Central Office for Research Ethics Committees (COREC)[14] issues guidelines for potential researchers wishing to conduct research on NHS patients and offers advice on the format of patient information sheets and consent forms.[17] Fig. 11.2 has been adapted to provide an example of an information sheet that could be used within veterinary practice for veterinary nursing research.

People should not feel in any way pressurised into taking part in a research study. There are occasions where people may feel obliged to take part, due to their relationship with the researcher.

Box 11.12

For example:
   A client has seen the same veterinary nurse with her pet for regular weight checks during the past year. This client, when approached by the veterinary nurse, may feel that she should agree to take part in the study as the veterinary nurse has always been 'so kind' to her dog.

A researcher needs to be aware of situations like this and where they perceive that there may be a problem, a third party, knowledgeable about the research that is due to take place, should be asked to obtain the person's informed consent.

All participants should be asked to sign a consent form prior to the commencement of a study. Fig. 11.1, adapted from a form issued by the Central Office for Research Ethics Committees,[14] provides an example that could be used in practice.

The principle of non-maleficence and the principle of beneficence

The principle of beneficence encompasses the sayings 'do good' and 'maximise possible benefits'. The principle of non-maleficence requires that the researcher 'avoids doing harm' to the participant. This is not always easy. Qualitative research, although not physically invasive, can be socially and emotionally invasive, thus having the potential to cause harm to the participants. That does not mean to say that research with the potential to 'harm' should not be conducted. However, it is important that the researcher addresses and assesses the risks of potential harm prior to the inception of a study, in order to maximise the benefits and reduce the risks.

A cost benefit analysis allows the researcher, and the research ethics committee, to make sure that the risks or costs of a study are commensurate with the benefit to society. The analysis takes into account all parties who may be involved in the study.

Participants and their families
There are many costs and benefits associated with being a research participant. It must be remembered, for example, that it can be damaging to be asked insensitive questions. A participant's confidence can be undermined, and they may be left feeling ignorant about a subject. The consequences of disclosing confidential information could have a huge impact on the participant and their family. However, participants often feel that by participating in a research study they have contributed to a worthwhile cause.

It is important that the researcher has the necessary skills to conduct the research, has been sufficiently trained in the research process and has the ability to phrase questions in a thoughtful and empathic way. Consent must be obtained prior to the start of the research. Participants should be given an information sheet detailing the advantages and disadvantages of the research prior to consent being given. Participants must be reassured that the information they provide will not be used against them.

Researchers

Researchers have to be aware that they may be harmed by conducting a research study. For example, they may uncover feelings of resentment towards clients or colleagues, or the research may rekindle previous personal negative experiences. However, the researcher may develop a greater understanding of a situation, thereby allowing them to reflect on their own thoughts and feelings, as well as obtaining results which may improve, for example, the quality of care given to an animal or client. The research may also contribute to a further qualification.

Researchers need to be aware of the ethical considerations behind the research they are conducting. It is easy for researchers to get 'carried away' with a thirst for knowledge and inadvertently violate ethical principles. Researchers need to address their own thoughts and feelings whilst conducting research and seek help and advice if required.

Investors

Research is an expensive undertaking. Investors provide funding which allows research to be conducted that might otherwise have been deemed too costly. However, there can be problems associated with research funding. It may be possible for the results to be biased. Although some investors may take an altruistic approach to sponsoring research, most investors sponsor research in the hope that the results will lead to increased profits, for example, by increasing the sales of a dressing material. This may put pressure on a researcher, especially if the research does not produce the expected results.

Researchers require intellectual honesty and integrity.

Society as a whole

Much research that is conducted has an effect on society as a whole. It is hoped that research will lead to an improved level of care and service. However, research that is carried out incorrectly could lead to the production of a biased and invalid set of results leading to a decline in care or incorrect information being produced.

Research should be conducted in a scientific, ethical manner. Biases, etc. should be minimised in order to produce a valid and reliable set of results. The results of research should be made available, even where these results are contrary to what was expected or hoped for.

The practice and practice staff

While it is hoped that practices will embrace veterinary nursing research as a way of improving patient and client care, it must be remembered that research can impede work, distract staff, create unrest and expose undesirable, unethical and questionable practice. Staff can become caught up in the ethical issues surrounding research without ever being actively involved, simply because they, their patients or clients become research participants. It is hoped that if the practice involves all staff in the research process from the start, the team will be more supportive and motivated, and will feel more positive about the results.

Box 11.13

A veterinary nurse wants to perform a piece of qualitative research within a practice to find out if clients within the practice are satisfied with the way their pets are admitted for surgery. She plans to interview them, using semi-structured interviews, within two days following the procedure.

Table 11.3 An example of some of the costs and benefits associated with this research proposal

	Cost	Benefit
Participants and their families	This piece of research could induce many emotions from the participant. Consider interviewing a client whose dog had to be euthanised on the operating table, or had died as the result of the anaesthetic or was experiencing post-operative complications. The emotions of guilt, depression, loneliness, sadness, etc. will be evident. This does not mean to say that these clients should not be part of the research as the experiences they had during the admission and consent process should have made them aware of the possible complications of both the anaesthetic and their involvement in the research. It is important that the researcher handles the situation professionally as the long-term effects to the client could be damaging.	The participants may feel a sense of gratitude in being able to discuss the situation with a friendly, impartial veterinary nurse. The participants may feel a sense of satisfaction at being able to provide information that may benefit others in the future.
Researchers	A sense of incompetence and unprofessionalism at not being able to deal with the distress a client may have suffered as a result of participation in the research.	A sense of achievement at having obtained results that will improve client care in the future.
Society as a whole		The publication of the results of this piece of research may help pet owners in general as improved admission procedures are adopted by veterinary practices.
Practice	The research may make the client aware that the admission procedure was not handled as it should have been giving rise to a client complaint. The researcher must not underestimate the fact that pet owners talk to each other outside the practice environment. This situation could therefore lead to bad publicity for the practice.	The improvement of client care and admission procedures.
To practice staff	May unearth problems related to the levels of competence and professionalism of certain staff within the practice. This in turn could lead to personnel problems if not addressed correctly.	May highlight areas of practice that need to be improved, and by addressing the areas of weakness within the practice team, improve client care long term by providing staff with appropriate further training. May improve job satisfaction.

CONCLUSION

Veterinary nurses are currently involved in research in a wide variety of ways, from being animal technicians and theatre nurses in scientific establishments, to being involved in and conducting clinical trials in veterinary practice. The knowledge and training that veterinary nurses have make them ideal candidates for these positions. It is anticipated that, within the next few years, veterinary nurses will not only be assisting with research studies, but will be conducting their own research studies and contributing to a knowledge base specific to the role of a veterinary nurse.

It is hoped that guidelines relating to the ethical review process will be produced, and the Guide to Professional Conduct for Veterinary Nurses will be rewritten, to include information for veterinary nurses wishing to be involved in the research process. Until that time, it is up to veterinary nurses to make sure that they consider the ethical and legal implications of all research proposals and studies, to ensure that veterinary nursing research is allowed to develop and establish itself as an integral part of the profession.

References

1. Jones JH. Bad blood: the Tuskegee syphilis experiment. In: Eckstein S. Manual for research ethics committees. 6th edn. Cambridge: Cambridge University Press; 2003.
2. Nicholson RH. The regulation of medical research: a historical overview. In: Eckstein S. Manual for research ethics committees. 6th edn. Cambridge: Cambridge University Press; 2003:19–20.
3. World Medical Association. Ethical principles for medical research involving human subjects (Declaration of Helsinki). In: Eckstein S. Manual for research ethics committees. 6th edn. Cambridge: Cambridge University Press; 2003:123–125.
4. The National Commission for the Protection of Human Subjects of Biomedical and Behavioural Research. The Belmont Report: Ethical principles and guidelines for the protection of human subjects of research. In: Eckstein S. Manual for research ethics committees. 6th edn. Cambridge: Cambridge University Press; 2003:126–132.
5. Department of Health. Governance arrangements for NHS research ethics committees. In: Eckstein S. Manual for research ethics committees. 6th edn. Cambridge: Cambridge University Press; 2003:150–163.
6. Lantra, Veterinary Nursing Manpower Survey; 2004.
7. Strauss A, Corbin J. Basics of qualitative research: grounded theory procedures and techniques. In: Holloway I, Wheeler S. Qualitative research for nurses; Oxford: Blackwell Science; 2000:2.
8. Porter S. Qualitative analysis. In: Cormack D. The research process in nursing. 4th edn. Oxford: Blackwell Science; 2000:399.
9. Holloway I, Wheeler S. Qualitative research for nurses; Oxford: Blackwell Science; 2000:78.
10. Beauchamp TL, Childress JE. Principles of biomedical ethics. Oxford: Oxford University Press; 1994.
11. Data Protection Act 1984. London: HMSO.
12. Pollit DF, Hungler BP. Essentials of nursing research methods, appraisal and utilization; 4th edn. Philadelphia: Lippincott Raven; 1997.
13. Royal College of Nursing. Research ethics: guidance for nurse involved in research or any investigative project involving human subjects. In: Eckstein S. Manual for research ethics committees. 6th edn. Cambridge: Cambridge University Press; 2003:260.
14. Central Office for Research Ethics Committees. Online. Available: http://www.corec.org.uk/ 19 Jan 2005.

12

A round-up of 'other' legislation

Carol Gray

The main legislation that currently affects veterinary nurses – animal welfare law, and the Veterinary Surgeons Act, has been covered in earlier chapters (see Chapters 6 and 9), but with what other animal-related legislation should the veterinary nurse be familiar? And what are the advantages of knowing something about animal law? Having a working knowledge of many different pieces of legislation can enhance job satisfaction (it increases confidence in your thoughts and actions), and will allow an exploration of the link between ethics and law. After all, it's one thing to work out your principles regarding 'difficult' situations on an ethical basis, but you also need to know the legal restrictions that apply.

By limiting this chapter to companion animals, including exotic species commonly presented as patients, it is possible to cover the subject under four main headings:

- Dangerous, exotic and wild animals.
- Sale of animals.
- Animal health and welfare.
- Civil law and liability.

DANGEROUS ANIMALS

Two main laws cover the ownership of dangerous animals: The Dangerous Dogs Act 1991[1] (and subsequent amendments 1997[2]), and the Dangerous Wild Animals Act 1976.[3]

The main difference between these statutes is the way in which the animals are licensed. The canine legislation requires the individual registration and fulfilment of attached conditions for each individual dog affected, whereas an application to keep other 'dangerous' animals requires the owner's premises to be licensed for the keeping of named numbers and species of animal.

Dangerous dogs

The Dangerous Dogs Act[1] (DDA) sets out certain conditions for the ownership of named breeds of dog, all recognised as fighting breeds. The main breed affected, in terms of numbers, was the American Pit Bull Terrier. As one of the requirements of the Act was the neutering of all registered Pit Bulls, it was hoped that the breed would die out in this country (indeed, that was the purpose of the Act). However, as this was a manufactured type of dog, it could easily be re-manufactured, and Pit Bull look-alikes are still seen in many parts of the country. They may appear in veterinary surgeries, un-muzzled, un-neutered and unregistered, with strange-sounding breed names (e.g., American Bulldog, Irish Staffordshire Bull Terrier).

So, the problem that became apparent with the original Act in the early 1990s, namely the difficulty of proving whether a dog was a Pit Bull Terrier or a Staffordshire Bull Terrier cross, is still apparent today. In the 'blitz' on Pit Bulls in the early days of the Act, the dogs were guilty until proven innocent (completely against the basic premise of the English legal system). Dogs were often held in custody for years, at great expense, while appeals were launched and 'behavioural experts' decided their fate.[4] Several high-profile cases hinged on minor points of law, for example, did the owner's car constitute a public place; did the removal of a registered dog's muzzle, to allow it to vomit, constitute an offence under the Act? In both cases, magistrates and judges decided they did. The dog in the car, Otis, was eventually condemned to death when appeals to the European Court of Human Rights failed on a technicality,[5] but the dog whose muzzle was removed, Dempsey, was reprieved after several appeals.[6]

This apparent unfairness led to the review of the Act in 1997, and the amendments included a correction of the most contentious part of the Act. This affected all breeds of dog, in that, if the owner was prosecuted under the DDA rather than older legislation (Dogs Act 1871[7]), the dog had to be killed if the offence was proved. Offences included being dangerously out of control in a public place, even if the dog did not actually bite anyone. No longer was every dog 'allowed one bite' as had been the case in the past. Again, there were several high-profile cases of dogs being sentenced to death in controversial circumstances, with many cases being taken to the appeal courts. One dog, Dino, was eventually reprieved in 2004, when the Criminal Cases Review Commission referred his case back to the Appeals Court, considering it to be a possible miscarriage of justice.[8] The 1997 amendments to the DDA allowed the magistrates/judges some discretion in sentencing, by ordering the means of control if a dog was not sentenced to death. For example, the owner may be ordered to have the dog neutered, to use a muzzle and have the dog on a lead when out in public.

Box 12.1

A client, sitting in the waiting room at a veterinary practice, is bitten on the leg by another client's dog, which is not on a lead.

According to the law, this is a public place, and if the client who is bitten reports the incident to the police, the owner may be prosecuted under the DDA, although this case may also be prosecuted under the older Dogs Act. Since the DDA amendment, the owner is more likely be obliged to carry out specific control measures than to have the dog seized and euthanased, as a defence may be the fact that the dog was stressed by the visit to the veterinary practice. As the dog was not on a lead,

the injured client could also bring a civil case for compensation against the dog's owner, if the bite wound is severe.

If the dog had been on a lead when it bit the other client, the outcome would be similar, in that the owner would be ordered to control the dog when in a public place. However, if the dog had not shown any aggressive tendencies before, it is unlikely that the owner could be sued by the injured party.

Box 12.2

The same dog is then being examined by the veterinary surgeon in a consulting room. He bites both the veterinary nurse and the owner.

It is accepted that the veterinary profession is responsible for employees' health and safety in the practice, and the vet should carry out a risk assessment on every dog that comes into the consulting room.[9] So in this case, the veterinary surgeon is liable, and the dog's owner is not to blame. (The waiting room is outwith the veterinary surgeon's control, as the dog has not yet been assessed). The veterinary nurse may well have a claim against the veterinary surgeon, as may the dog's owner. In fact, many practices in the USA now refuse to allow clients to handle their own animals for examination or treatment, and insist on this being done by veterinary technicians (their equivalent of veterinary nurses).

Guard dogs

What about keeping a dog specifically for protection? For protection of premises other than a residential dwelling, the dog must be restrained to prevent it roaming free, or be under the constant control of the handler (Guard Dogs Act 1975[10]). Signs must alert visitors to the presence of guard dogs. A dog kept for protection at home, which bites a visitor or intruder, may fall foul of the legislation for dangerous dogs.

Other dangerous animals

Other animals that are considered to be a danger to the public (if allowed to roam free) are listed under the Dangerous Wild Animals Act 1976,[3] which imposes licensing conditions on the keepers of such animals. Common species, which require licences under this Act, include all wild cats, wild dogs and wolves. Licences are granted following inspections carried out by a veterinary surgeon on behalf of the Local Authority. Two fairly common 'pet' breeds governed by the DWA Act are the wolf hybrid and the Bengal cat. These were added to the list of dangerous animals in modification Orders.[11]

This followed public pressure in response to several high-profile stories of humans injured by wolf hybrids. The problem here, as with Pit Bull Terriers, is proving whether an individual animal is a true wolf hybrid or a husky-type crossbreed. The only definitive method of proof is via DNA testing, which is expensive, and may not give a definitive answer (see below). Under the terms of the Act, any wolf hybrid (for many generations from the original cross) will require a licence, and cannot be taken out in public places.

The Bengal cat is a cross between the Asian leopard cat (*Felis bengalensis*, a wild cat, which definitely requires a DWA licence) and the domestic cat (*Felis catus*, mainly using the Egyptian Mau, Abyssinian and Ocicat breeds). Most Bengal cats in this country are now at least four generations from the original wild cat, but many local authorities are insistent that any Bengal cats require a DWA licence, using similar grounds to those used for the wolf hybrids. Others will only insist on licensing if the cats are from the first few generations below the wild ancestor. There seems to be a problem with consistency among local authorities. DNA testing would probably not help in this case, as many genes would be common to both species, but accurate pedigree recording may help to prove the generational relationship to wild ancestors. The main challenge to the law seems to be on the behaviour and characteristics of the animal concerned. If an individual does not show the species-specific behaviour and appearance of an excluded animal (i.e. a domestic dog or cat), then it requires a licence. Expert witnesses can often disagree, however, on an interpretation of 'species-specific' behaviour. A civil case ruling, that a dog with less than 1 per cent wolf genes could not be classified as *Canis familiaris* (domestic dog), set a precedent for any future cases in this area.[12]

EXOTIC ANIMALS

Veterinary nurses who work to any great extent with exotic animals require a working knowledge of the relevant legislation.

CITES (Convention on International Trade in Endangered Species of Wild Flora and Fauna – 1973)[13]

The main law governing the keeping of exotic animals is the Endangered Species (Import and Export) Act 1976,[14] which enforces the principles of the CITES agreement in this country. The CITES agreement limits international trade in animals and plants, with licensing conditions for species listed in the Convention being dependent on the status of the species in the wild. Most exotic pets are now bred here, and therefore do not come under the terms of this Act, but any new species presented may raise concerns about wild capture and illegal importation.

All tortoises should now be bred in this country. If there is any doubt, CITES documents should be produced to confirm that the animal has been legally obtained. Is it your duty to check this? Certainly it should be the responsibility of the veterinary surgeon who sees the animal, and correct identification of the species will be required for the consent form.

Drug treatment

The other main area of concern is the drugs used for treatment of these species. Very few drugs are licensed for use in exotic animals. Most practices that specialise in exotic animals will have standard

---

Box 12.3

A client has brought in a 'new' species of tortoise that you have never seen before – and they are slightly evasive about how/where they acquired it.

---

consent forms, allowing use of non-licensed products, which clients must sign before any treatment is given. This must be informed consent, so the clients must be made aware of the risks involved in using non-licensed products on their animals.

WILD ANIMALS

Rehabilitation

Well-meaning members of the public often bring injured or diseased wild animals into veterinary practices, but when should such creatures be rehabilitated? Many species are now covered by the Wildlife and Countryside Act 1981,[15] which affords different levels of protection to certain species of bird, and to some native wild animals. Birds of prey receive the highest level of protection. It is illegal to remove eggs or young birds, or to disturb nests, of named species. Any fledglings brought into the practice should be carefully identified and returned to where they were found, if possible. There are exceptions to the law when it comes to birds requiring veterinary treatment; even birds given the highest level of protection can be cared for in captivity until fully recovered, but must then be released if capable of surviving in the wild.

An ethical dilemma occurs if an animal is too badly injured to be re-released. Is it fair to attempt treatment if it is destined to spend the rest of its life in captivity? If full recovery is anticipated, it may be interesting for the vets and nurses involved to try some 'experimental' treatment on an unusual patient, or to try to provide nursing care in a practice. What about the stress experienced by the patient during treatment? It is subjected to close human contact, to other animals including predators, and to an unusual environment. Is the outcome sufficiently beneficial to justify the means? One option might be to refer the animal to a specialist wildlife hospital, where its environmental needs may be better provided for.

Re-release of non-native species

Another common legal problem arises with the rescue of injured non-native wildlife. According to the WCA, they can never be re-released into the wild. Species involved include the grey squirrel, Canada goose, red-eared terrapin and even the budgerigar!

Box 12.4
A client has brought in a grey squirrel, which has been injured in a road accident. It is mildly concussed, with an obvious hind-limb fracture.

Even if the client agrees that they will take the animal home after treatment, and keep it in captivity for the rest of its life, is it fair to condemn the animal to this sort of future? What if you suspect that the client intends to re-release the squirrel? Should you refuse to give it back? Or is it the client's decision whether to break the law? This may be a dilemma that requires the veterinary surgeon to take ultimate responsibility, but it is a situation that lends itself to the formulation of a practice policy on injured non-native wildlife. This will allow all members of the practice team to voice their opinions, and to be involved in the process.

SALE OF ANIMALS

Nothing brings home the status of animals in law quite as profoundly as the legislation governing buying and selling animals. The view of animals as the owner's 'goods' or 'property' means that the Sale of Goods Act 1979 (SGA)[16] applies just as well to the sale of an animal as to the sale of an electric toaster.

Greatest protection is given to the buyer in a business sale. With private sales, the saying 'caveat emptor' (buyer beware) applies. The only legal obligation for the private seller is that he/she must have the right to sell, that is, that the animal is theirs to sell, and has not been stolen.

Box 12.5
A horse owner has loaned a horse to a friend. This person sells the horse without the owner's permission.

Here, it may seem apparent that the seller has committed an offence under the Theft Act 1968,[17] but there may be a problem proving ownership. Did the horse's original owner 'give' the horse to their friend, or was a proper loan agreement drawn up, detailing the conditions of the loan? In either case, it is probably the end of the friendship!

In business sales, the protection extends to the animal matching the description given by the seller, being fit for its intended purpose, and being of 'satisfactory quality'. This means that animals bought from dealers or pet shops (where the vendor sells animals in the course of a business) are covered by the SGA. However, there is one important exception to this. The provisions that animals must be 'fit for purpose' and be of 'satisfactory quality' only apply if the opinion of an expert has *not* been sought. This means that if someone buys a horse from a dealer without having a pre-purchase examination carried out by a veterinary surgeon, they will have full legal protection should the horse turn out to have a problem. If, however, they have a pre-purchase examination carried out, it becomes the veterinary surgeon's responsibility. It is the veterinary surgeon who will suffer the financial consequences, if the examination fails to reveal conditions that may affect the horse's value or fitness for purpose. The vet who carried out the pre-purchase examination may be liable for the difference in value between the horse when it was bought (apparently without any problems), and a horse with the condition that the examination failed to reveal. With small animals, where performance is not such a big issue, things are not quite so clear.

Box 12.6

A family bought a labrador pup as a pet, from a large pet superstore. The dog became lame at five months old, and was eventually diagnosed as having hip dysplasia, probably a hereditary condition. On investigation by the family, it turned out that the pup's parents did not have hip x-rays taken and scored before they were mated. Do the family have a case against the pet store?

In terms of the Sale of Goods Act, yes they do . . . they bought the pup from a commercial dealer, as a family pet. If it is chronically lame, it cannot fulfil that purpose. They did not have the pup checked by an independent expert before they bought it, so they have full protection under the law. However, under the terms of the SGA, they should have returned the pup within a reasonable time (usually 30 days) for a full refund, but the condition did not show up until the pup was five months old, a common age for this condition to become apparent.

What can the family do? They could offer the pet store a chance to make things better, for example, by paying for any surgical operations to sort out the condition, in order to allow the pup to live a comfortable life. However, this is likely to add up to an amount far in excess of the price paid for the pup. They could ask for a refund of all, or part of, the purchase price. This would mean that the family could keep the pup, to whom they have become very attached, but the seller would make some contribution to veterinary fees. The seller may offer to replace the pup with another one. This would probably be the cheapest option for the seller, but would be totally unacceptable to the family. This case illustrates the difference between animals and electric toasters!

The sale of dogs is also governed by the Breeding and Sale of Dogs (Welfare) Act 1999,[18] which was intended to eliminate puppy farms. This Act puts the onus on licensed breeders to sell only to licensed pet stores, and to correctly identify all puppies sold with a collar and identity tag. It is intended that this piece of legislation should be incorporated into the proposed Animal Welfare Bill.[19]

Some animal sales require more stringent contracts between buyer and seller. For example, the sale of Specified Pathogen Free (SPF) animals for research, or animals with a specific genetic make-up, requires a very clear description of the animals involved. The SPF or genetic status of the animals is regarded as a 'condition' of sale, and breaches of a condition of sale are regarded as very serious. In this case, the buyer would be entitled to a full refund. Few other animal sales involve conditions of sale.

Less important characteristics are referred to as 'warranties' and these are often involved in commercial horse sales. A warranty may guarantee freedom from vices, for example. Should the horse turn out to have a vice, the buyer will be entitled to a refund of the difference between the price paid and the horse's actual value. Most horses bought from horse sales will be 'warranted' free from vices such as crib-biting and weaving.

Business sales are policed by Trading Standards Officers, who regularly visit places where animals are sold, to ensure that they are operating within the law. They also investigate complaints from buyers.

Having looked at the legal situation, it would seem that if someone is going to spend a large amount of money on an animal, they should buy from a commercial dealer, as they will have more protection in law. This contradicts traditional advice that it is best to buy pedigree animals from small-scale breeders, and to see the sire and dam. What is the best advice to give to clients? It would seem that if 'performance' is important, then it is preferable to buy from a commercial dealer. A private sale, in this case, should rely on the opinion of an expert (i.e. a veterinary surgeon), who will charge for this, but who will then take on the burden of financial responsibility should their opinion be incorrect. If buying an animal for companionship, then the opportunity to examine both parents will give a likely indication of future size, health, looks and temperament. This would point the buyer towards a private sale, as it is unusual to have this opportunity with commercial sellers.

ANIMAL HEALTH AND WELFARE

Prevention of disease

In general, veterinary nurses will not be involved in procedures to prevent notifiable disease. They should be aware that DEFRA (Department for the Environment, Food and Rural Affairs) maintains vigilance, by means of a list of animal diseases (mainly affecting farm livestock) which must be reported to them if diagnosed. Orders for notifiable disease control are made under the Animal Health Act 1981.[20] The notifiable disease of most interest to veterinary nurses is rabies; because of this disease, the import and export of cats and dogs is strictly controlled. Recently, alternatives to quarantine have been available, such as the Pet Travel Scheme.[21] The downside to easier international travel for dogs and cats is the possibility of the introduction of new exotic diseases. A voluntary reporting scheme (DACTARI – Dog and Cat Travel and Risk Information) has been set up to monitor cases of exotic disease in dogs and cats.[22]

Companion animals can become involved in the control measures for notifiable diseases. For example, in the 2001 Foot and Mouth Disease epidemic in the United Kingdom, many footpaths were closed to people and dogs. Horse owners were also affected, with bridleways closed, and horse events initially suspended. In the case of a rabies outbreak, cats and dogs must be confined indoors, or kept strictly under control (muzzled and on a lead).[23]

Animal health legislation also includes transport of animals, with maximum journey times for all species of livestock. The Welfare of Animals (Transport) Order 1995[24] was introduced to enact a European Union Directive, and applies to all vertebrate animals. However, pet cats and dogs are excluded if travelling with the owner, and horses are only included if they are not travelling for the purposes of competition.

Identification of animals

Are you sure that the dog is the individual that the client says it is?

Identification of animals is governed by various pieces of legislation. For example, dogs registered under the Dangerous Dogs Act are required to be tattooed AND microchipped. All farm animals must be permanently identified by ear tags.[25] Horses must be clearly identified on their passports,

---

Box 12.7

A client who breeds black Labradors has brought in one of her young dogs for a BVA/KC Hip Dysplasia Scheme hip x-ray. The dog is identified only by means of a collar and ID tag. She has ten dogs, and has had trouble with hip dysplasia in her lines in the past.

a requirement for every equine.[26] Dogs and cats being taken out of the country must be micro-chipped as a condition of the Pet Travel Scheme. However, there is no requirement (at the moment) to permanently identify dogs and cats that do not come under the categories above.

All dogs must wear a collar and identity tag when out in a public place[27] but there is no require-ment to have collars on cats.

In the above scenario, the client may only have a few dogs, which are regular patients at the practice, and therefore well known to practice staff. However, it may be that the client has a large number of dogs, tends to use several practices, and there may be some doubt about the identity of the animal presented for the BVA/KC health scheme involved.

Other licences required for keeping animals

The welfare of animals kept in business establish-ments is governed by the requirement for licences for the owners of these businesses. Therefore, owners of boarding establishments for dogs and cats,[28] breeding establishments for dogs,[29] pet shops[30] and riding establishments[31] require licences from the Local Authority. Veterinary surgeons are involved in the inspection of riding establish-ments, and may be asked to be involved in other inspections, but officers from the Local Authority (environmental health department) are usually responsible for the rest. It is intended to include legislation for these licences in the new Animal Welfare Bill.

CIVIL LAW AND LIABILITY FOR ANIMALS

Responsibility for animals, and any damage that they cause, is dependent on species (Animals Act 1971[32]). Owners of dangerous wild animals or dan-gerous dogs have 'strict' liability for any damage done to persons or property. This means that they are wholly responsible for the consequences of the animal's actions (hence the need to have third party insurance for dogs that may bite). Damages awarded are usually high, as the dangerous animal should not have been allowed to roam.

Damage done by any dog is still the responsibil-ity of the owner. Dogs that cause road accidents, or injure other dogs, cats or humans, will cost their owners a large amount of money, whether for car repair, human injury claims or veterinary treat-ment. Dogs should be under their owners' control at all times. If a dog strays on to farmland and injures or kills livestock, the farmer is entitled to kill or injure the dog if that is the only way to stop it. This must be reported to a police station within 48 hours.[32] Pet insurance schemes include third party insurance as part of their policies. Owners are not responsible for damage done to people or property by cats (except for those cats that require Dangerous Wild Animals licences). In general, it is recognised that owners have no control over cats. A driver who swerves to avoid a cat running across the road, and crashes into another car, will have to make a claim on his car insurance. The cat owner has no legal liability.

However, cats are regarded as their owner's property.

Box 12.8

A client has brought in a male cat for neutering, claiming that it is her cat. It subsequently transpires that it is her neighbour's cat, which she has 'kidnapped' in order to have the operation carried out, to prevent him fighting with her own cat.

The neighbour could sue this client for trespass, as she has interfered with their 'goods'. There would be no blame attached to the veterinary prac-tice, which carried out the operation in good faith (obviously, the client signed the consent form fraudulently as the owner or the 'owner's agent'), but this could turn into an unpleasant case for the veterinary practice to be involved with. Members of staff may be called as witnesses for the plaintiff (the person bringing the case) in a civil court case.

CONCLUSION

In summary, a working knowledge of the law can enhance the veterinary nurse's role in practice. For example, it may make giving advice to clients easier. Ethical principles should underlie the law-making process, but in many of the examples given, there seems to be a conflict between what is ethically desirable, and what is legally permissible. Ethics are what an individual uses to make personal decisions in a given situation, but knowledge of the legal background to the situation is required to rule out any 'ethical' choices that are outside the law.

References

1. Dangerous Dogs Act 1991. London: HMSO.
2. Dangerous Dogs (Amendment) Act 1997. London: HMSO.
3. Dangerous Wild Animals Act 1976. London: HMSO.
4. Radford M. Animal welfare law in Britain – regulation and responsibility. Oxford: Oxford University Press; 2001:348.
5. Bates v. UK, ECHR, 16 Jan 1996.
6. R v. Ealing Justices ex parte Fanneran, QBD, 9 Dec 1995.
7. Dogs Act 1871. London: HMSO.
8. R v. Northampton Crown Court ex parte Lamont, Criminal Cases Review Commission 302/04; 15 Oct 2004.
9. Health and Safety at Work Act 1974. London: HMSO.
10. Guard Dogs Act 1975. London: HMSO.
11. Dangerous Wild Animals Act 1976 Modification Orders 1981, 1984. London: HMSO.
12. Wildin v. Rotherham Metropolitan Borough Council 1997.
13. Convention on International Trade in Endangered Species of Wild Fauna and Flora 1973 (Washington Convention; CITES). Online. Available: http://www.cites.org/eng/disc/text.shtml 19 May 2005.
14. Endangered Species (Import and Export) Act 1976. London: HMSO.
15. Wildlife and Countryside Act 1981. London: HMSO.
16. Sale of Goods Act 1979. London: HMSO.
17. Theft Act 1968. London: HMSO.
18. Breeding and Sale of Dogs (Welfare) Act 1999. London: HMSO.
19. Draft Animal Welfare Bill, July 2004. London: TSO.
20. Animal Health Act 1981. London: HMSO.
21. Department for the Environment, Food and Rural Affairs. Pet travel scheme. Online. Available: http://www.defra.gov.uk/animalh/quarantine/pets/index.htm 9 May 2005.
22. Department for the Environment, Food and Rural Affairs. Dog and cat travel and risk information. Online. Available: http://www.defra.gov.uk/animalh/diseases/veterinary/dactari/index.htm. 9 May 2005.
23. Rabies (Control) Order 1974. London: HMSO.
24. Welfare of Animals (Transport) Order 1995. London: HMSO.
25. Cattle Identification Regulations 1998, Council Regulation (EC) No. 21/2004.
26. Horse Passports (England) Regulations 2004. London: HMSO.
27. Control of Dogs Order 1992, SI 1992/901. London: HMSO.
28. Animal Boarding Establishments Act 1963. London: HMSO.
29. Breeding of Dogs Act 1973. London: HMSO.
30. Pet Animals Act 1951. London: HMSO.
31. Riding Establishments Act 1970. London: HMSO.
32. Animals Act 1971. London: HMSO.

13

Ethical thinking: the way forward?

Dympna Crowley

Perhaps the way forward for the veterinary nursing profession is to consider a parallel body, that of human nursing. Reflecting on the developments and achievements of human nurses should give some insight as to what lies ahead for veterinary nurses. The similarities between the two groups are obvious. Human nursing developed in response to a need by society and the medical profession. It was originally based on the 'apprentice' system of training. The emphasis now on education, as opposed to training, and a move into higher education is creating a knowledgeable body of professionals who can think and act for themselves. They are confident both in themselves and their ability to deliver professional nursing care. This growing confidence comes with the knowledge that human nursing is seen by society as a profession.

Veterinary nursing is needed by society and veterinarians to care for animals. Veterinary nurses are now educated in higher education, both to degree level and through the Advanced Diploma in Veterinary Nursing. There is a strong motivation towards professionalism and to be seen to be professionals in practice. However, professionalism is more than a label. It is inseparable from ethical, lawful and accountable practice. To function as professionals, veterinary nurses need to explore and analyse what it means to be a professional. This chapter will focus on some of the key concepts associated with professionalism with an emphasis on ethical professionalism.

WHAT IS A PROFESSION?

This term is used by many occupations today. We have professional footballers, professional musicians and so on. Originally medicine and law were called professions. Nowadays it can be used to describe an occupation whose members are required to have a 'degree of skill and specific knowledge'.[1] An earlier exploration by Carr-Saunders and Wilson in 1964[2] stated that the term profession '. . . clearly stands for something. That something is a complex of characteristics'. However, they did not establish what these characteristics are. Many writers have attempted to do this, and have come up with lists that can be considered to describe a profession, but agreement is not uniform. Within human nursing, the characteristics compiled by Hall,[3] which are taken from several lists, are still used today as a backdrop to the debate.

Box 13.1 The characteristics of a profession

1. It provides a service to society, involving specialised knowledge and skills.
2. It possesses a unique body of knowledge, which it constantly seeks to extend in order to improve its service.
3. It educates its own practitioners.
4. It sets its own standards.
5. It adapts its services to meet changing needs.
6. It accepts responsibility for safeguarding the public it serves.
7. It strives to make economical use of its practitioners.
8. It promotes the welfare and well-being of its practitioners and safeguards their interests.
9. It is motivated more by its commitment to the service it renders than by considerations of economic gain.

---

10. It adheres to a code of conduct based on ethical principles.
11. It unites for strength in achieving its larger purposes.
12. It is self-governing.

These characteristics are revisited and revised frequently. While the debate continues as to whether human nursing is a profession or not, the current consensus is that it is a profession, albeit an emerging one.

The list of characteristics helps to distinguish a profession from an occupation. In addition, members of a profession are usually registered with a recognisable body. In human nursing this is the Nursing and Midwifery Council. The NMC is the nursing and midwifery regulatory body. It is required by statute law to establish and improve standards of nursing and midwifery care in order to protect the public. The standards are set out in the Code of Professional Conduct.[4] Since August 2004 the title of this code has been extended; it is now The NMC code of professional conduct: standards for conduct, performance and ethics.[5] The NMC maintains a register of licensed practitioners. These practitioners have reached a satisfactory level of competence and have a suitable character, which is usually verified by the university or college they have attended.[6]

In relating these characteristics to veterinary nursing, it is worth recalling that human nursing is a young profession, and as such, does not demonstrate all of the characteristics to the same extent as the long established professions like medicine and law.[3] As far back as the early 1970s, a major report commissioned by the government described nursing as 'the major caring profession' and the claim was justified because nursing reflected many of the characteristics of a profession.[3] Thirty years on, this debate continues, in spite of the developments towards professionalism. Human nursing is now considered to be a profession, albeit an evolving or emerging one. One possible reason for this is that, although nursing is recognised as a profession in the UK, USA and South Africa, in many countries this process has just started, while in others no attempt has been made to professionalise

it.[6] To seek and earn professional status, any group pursuing this aim should exhibit the characteristics associated with professional conduct.

Professionalism is inextricably linked to ethical conduct. An analysis of the literature will show that being a professional carries with it important ethical implications.[8] This is due largely to the term 'professional' being essentially a social concept. Society decides that it needs the knowledge, skills and expertise of a group of individuals whose work is complex and necessary. This creates a social contract. The public expects the profession to honour its obligation, to continually monitor and evaluate its practice, and to deal with members who are unprofessional. This gives professions privileged status. Professionals are valued by society. They are needed and rewarded financially. Essentially, society endorses a profession. However, if the profession reneges on its obligations, society can be damning in its retribution. It is worth remembering that the actions of a few can jeopardise the reputations of all involved.[9] The conduct of individual nurses can, all too often, give the profession a bad press. The recent cases of human nurses assisting the deaths of older people in their care bring this into sharp focus. The public confidence in human nursing is maintained by the action of the profession in dealing with such nurses.

Professionals are valued for their contribution to society. They are seen to have integrity, and respect for the professional–client relationship is paramount. Underpinning this is their commitment to respect fundamental professional values. These values are what attract individuals to the profession, and members of society to seek their assistance. This is endorsed by an additional and more recently published characteristic. 'A profession is distinguished by the presence of a specific culture, norms, and values that are common among its members.'[10]

PROFESSIONAL VALUES AND THE NEED TO CLARIFY THEM

Veterinary practice is diverse. One practice may be set up to care for domestic animals, another for farm animals, another for exotic animals and so on. It is suggested that veterinary medicine is more diverse and complex than human medicine.[11] This diversity reflects how animals are valued within society. For example, we may value animals as pets, as a source of food or as both, but when it comes to professional veterinary practice, these values should be ethically sound.

Ethics can be considered to be the study of what is valued by humans in their conduct with others, including animals. This explores how humans relate to others, and their conduct is scrutinised to establish if their behaviour is good or bad, right or wrong. One of the hallmarks of a profession is that its members are ethical in their professional practice. To develop as a profession, it is necessary to look critically at the key values of the profession. This is often called values clarification. It is not a one-off exercise. From time to time, it needs to be revisited and revised to keep abreast of developments and changes in practice.

As individuals, human beings have moral values and make moral judgments. They express them and sometimes discuss them. For example, an individual may have an opinion about environmental issues. When this is expressed, it gives others an insight into the values that underpin this opinion. This facilitates a discussion with those who share this opinion or hold opposing views. This may be viewed as moralising; however, it is, in fact, ethics. The following example illustrates the difference.

Box 13.2

If I say it is wrong to tell a lie, this is moralising. If I am concerned with why it is wrong to tell a lie, this is ethics, as I am considering the judgement itself, its significance, its underlying value, and not solely the behaviour.

Values are dynamic. They change and develop through personal and professional experiences.[12] It is acknowledged that a person's character is defined by their value choices, which in turn develop their value system, and are expressed in their value judgements.[13]

In professional practice it is often unclear what is valued.

Box 13.3

For example, a veterinary nurse may be uncertain about euthanasing a healthy animal, docking the tail of a puppy or aggressively treating an old and very sick cat.

It is essential that veterinary nurses are clear about what they value. In a profession like veterinary nursing, which is animal- and person-centred, the integration of these values into their professional practice influences society's concept of the profession and the quality of care given.[14]

Clarification of values can help sort out those that are worth keeping and those that are not. This is done through analysis and prioritisation of values that are consistent with ethical veterinary nursing practice. Professional values are beliefs and attitudes about the worth of the profession. They guide behaviour and endorse standards of conduct that are professionally acceptable. Values form the basis of actions. If time is not taken to examine and articulate values, it is likely that the relationship between the professional, the patient and the client is not fully effective. Veterinary nurses need to be clear about what they value, in order to choose and initiate a course of action that is consistent with what they believe in, and is professionally acceptable.

Box 13.4

For example, a veterinary nurse who values honesty will aim to be honest with her colleagues, clients and herself.

The price paid for unexamined values is that there may be a conflict of values and interests. This leads to confusion and inconsistency in the decision-making process and resulting actions.[15]

There are several ways of clarifying values. The simplest method is to list values that are at the heart of veterinary nursing practice, analyse them and put them in order of priority. This approach to the evaluation of ethical and moral issues was developed during the 1960s,[16] when steps in the process were identified. It is suggested that values are confirmed when the following are achieved:

- Choosing freely.
- Choosing from alternatives.
- Choosing after considering the consequences.
- Cherishing the choice.
- Publicly affirming the value.
- Acting consistently on the chosen value.

Box 13.5

For example, in selecting honesty, the veterinary nurse has made a choice, considered the alternative (which is to be deceitful) and taken the consequences into account. She publicly displays this choice by being honest with colleagues, clients and herself.

A veterinary nurse will probably choose to work in a veterinary practice based on her own value system. That choice could be influenced by the focus of a particular practice.

Box 13.6

For example, a veterinary nurse has chosen to work with farm animals, but realises that this area of the profession is more concerned with the economic value of the animals, rather than the animals themselves.

While working as an employee, there is the possibility that from time to time there will be a conflict of values. It is important to examine the nature of the conflict and consider if the difficulty is related to personal or professional values. This should help to clarify what is at a stake. In veterinary nursing practice, the frame of reference to use is the RCVS Guide to Professional Conduct for Veterinary Nurses.

THE LINK BETWEEN VALUES AND ETHICS

Veterinary nurses encounter all sorts of situations in veterinary practice that will make them ask questions. There reactions will depend on their experience, knowledge of similar situations and values. These values may be challenged and called into question. Difficulties faced may involve an apparent disregard for fundamental values. However, colleagues may not share these values. To establish fundamental professional values, the ethical principles established by contemporary philosophical writers can be used. Table 13.1 gives examples of how ethical principles may support values in practice.

PROFESSIONAL ACCOUNTABILITY

In the early 1980s, the United Kingdom Central Council (UKCC) introduced accountability into

Table 13.1

Ethical principles Beauchamp, Childress[17] and Gillon[18]	Ethical principles Thiroux[19]	How values are related to practice
Autonomy	The value of life, honesty	Animals are respected and the 'five freedoms' are promoted. Clients are informed and told the truth
Beneficence	Goodness or rightness	Animal welfare is promoted and the client benefits from the professional advice given
Non-maleficence	To cause no harm or badness	Actual and potential harms to the animal are discussed with the client, and animal welfare is promoted
Justice	Fairness	The quality of the time given to each animal and client is equal

human nursing, in its first code of conduct. This was swiftly followed by various UKCC documents that endorsed the concept. Up until this time, nurses were seen as mainly responsible for their actions. What this meant was that nurses were given tasks or duties, such as patient care, for which they were answerable. When this was done, the responsibility ceased. In the event of something going wrong, the buck was passed further up the nursing hierarchy. This practice can be traced back to the early years of nursing, when nurses were trained rather than educated.[20] The apprenticeship system of training encouraged obedience, that is, following orders.[21] The introduction of professional accountability required nurses to think, and to recognise that the buck now stopped with them.

Professionalism and accountability go hand in hand. Veterinary nursing is not yet regulated and, therefore, not seen as profession. Hopefully, it is moving towards professional regulation. Once a body is established, and it is seen as a profession, its members are accountable. This process can be challenging and complex, but it is inescapable.

To understand professional accountability, veterinary nurses could use the NMC code of professional conduct[5] as a frame of reference. Nurses and midwives are reminded repeatedly in the code that they are personally accountable for their practice. The introduction to the code makes is quite clear that personal accountability means 'that you are answerable for your actions and omissions, regardless of advice or directions from another professional'.[5]

Box 13.7

A nurse who delegates an aspect of care to another nurse is accountable for that aspect of care which has been delegated, whereas the nurse who delivers the aspect of care is responsible for doing it.

Accountability is 'responsibility for something or someone'.[5] It seems that accountability and responsibility mean the same and are used interchangeably. Within human nursing, an analysis of the concept recognises this, but a distinction is made between accountability and responsibility professionally.[22] The difference is important.

A nurse is both responsible and accountable for patient care. 'While responsibility is a key component of accountability it is only a part of it. Accountability is more inclusive than responsibility'.[23] Accountability is ongoing and can be considered to being like a cyclical process. It requires a situation to be assessed, a plan to be made and carried out and the results evaluated. Responsibility refers to a task, and when the task has been done, the responsibility ceases. Accountability requires a nurse to be responsible but responsibility does not assume accountability.[24]

Accountability and responsibility is not just the domain of nurses in direct contact with patients and clients. Those in a managerial position are also under an obligation to accept that their role requires them to be both accountable and responsible. In reality nurses in senior positions who renege on their responsibilities in this area are likely to suffer the consequences for their actions or omissions.

Box 13.8

A senior veterinary nurse in a busy practice had managerial responsibility for the theatre area where she worked with two other veterinary nurses. One of these nurses was on long-term sick leave, leaving her to work with the less experienced nurse. The senior veterinary nurse was very conscientious and hard working and considered to be very reliable. One day the practice manager found her staggering around the unit. When asked what was wrong she admitted to taking some amphetamines which she got from a friend. She said that these help her to cope with the increased demands of managing the theatre. The stress she was experiencing was caused by the acceptance that she was considered to be capable and reliable, and she did not want to admit to not being able to cope.

On the one hand, this veterinary nurse would seem to be unprofessional. She should acknowledge the limitations of her ability. On the other hand, she may have a very committed approach to being a professional, in that she has to work above and beyond the call of duty. While this may be the case, the practice manager has failed to manage the situation appropriately, by assuming that the veterinary nurse could cope, and not replacing the veterinary nurse on long-term sick leave. This situation could be seen as a wake up call in that this incident did not affect any patient, client or colleague. Had her drug-taking not been discovered, there could have been far-reaching professional, legal and ethical consequences.

This scenario also highlights that being accountable can be problematic. Many writers have questioned whether it is possible to be accountable without having authority.[21] It is suggested that responsibility and authority are necessary for accountability to be exercised. It would seem to be inappropriate to hold a veterinary nurse accountable for resources over which she has no control. In this scenario she is professionally accountable, as she has not stated that she cannot cope with the reduction in staffing levels. She is not responsible for staffing the theatre, so she cannot be held accountable for not replacing the veterinary nurse who is on long-term sick leave, as she does not have the authority to do so. However, her practice manager is accountable, as she has the authority to replace the veterinary nurse who is on long-term sick leave.

This distinction between accountability and responsibility is useful when explaining levels of accountability to students.

Accountability is earned through education, experience and professional development. Students of any profession have to learn knowledge, skills and attitudes, and develop fundamental values applicable to the profession. These are considered to be the preconditions of accountability.[23]

Box 13.9

Pre-registration human nursing students are not accountable in the same way as registered nurses. Registered nurses are professionally accountable for the actions or omissions of the students they supervise. This is why students must be supervised in practice. This does not mean that students can never be called to account by their university or by law for the consequences of their actions or omissions.[5]

Once registered, a nurse is professionally accountable. Within health and veterinary care, nurses work with other registered professionals. They are, in turn, professionally accountable for their areas of practice. There are role boundaries, but in practice they may not always be clearly drawn.

ETHICAL ACCOUNTABILITY

Accountability within human nursing has been discussed and debated for over three decades. The evolution of accountability is linked to how society expects professionals to behave and conduct themselves, and the need to audit and explain public expenditure.[23] Society invests in health professionals' education and training, and the professionals are expected to deliver health care when it is needed. Should professionals fall short in their delivery, society will hold them to account. The Kennedy Report 2001[25] is a powerful reminder of the consequences of unprofessional conduct.

There is a moral dimension to professional accountability. Choosing to enter a profession, and completing the education, training, and assessments required, is a personal achievement. The personal and professional investment is enormous. This investment must be respected by the individual, as well as by the profession.

Consumers of health care are better educated and informed, and expect to be involved in deci-

Box 13.10

This report followed the inquiry into children's heart surgery at Bristol Royal Infirmary. The clinicians connected with pediatric cardiac services had data highlighting their poor performance and high mortality rate, relative to other centres in the UK. They did not stop to reflect and question why this might be, but continued their work. The report criticised named healthcare professionals, including medical and nursing personnel, for poor management, and a lack of leadership and insight. Some were regarded as having failed to treat patients with respect and honesty.

sions about their treatment and care. They also have an expectation of how a professional should relate to them. Health care in general, and nursing in particular, is moving towards increasing openness and transparency within the profession.

Box 13.12

For example, a veterinary surgeon may focus on the current welfare of the animal, while the veterinary nurse may also be concerned about the future welfare of the animal.

Box 13.11

For example, a registered human nurse advised a patient with a urinary tract infection to drink cranberry juice. She stated that there was no clear evidence that it worked, but her experience, and anecdotal evidence, indicated that it did. This left the decision, whether to drink cranberry juice or not, with the patient. This promotes respect for patients' autonomy.

Box 13.13

For example, a veterinary nurse could advocate for a change in practice policy, from one that will perform spaying operations on pregnant cats, to one that promotes early neutering of female kittens.

THE VETERINARY NURSE'S PROFESSIONAL RELATIONSHIPS

Many different groups will look critically at how veterinary nurses conduct themselves.[26] Firstly, veterinary nursing practice is a tripartite relationship (between the patient, the client and the veterinary nurse). Secondly, veterinary nurses are usually employees, so there is an additional relationship between the veterinary nurse and the employer. Thirdly, there is also a relationship between veterinary nursing practice and society, which includes ordinary citizens, consumers, government, animal protectionists and so on. These groups look critically at how veterinary nurses do their job and deal with their professional responsibilities.

As previously stated, professionalism is inextricably linked to ethical conduct and practice. This applies equally to all the veterinary nurse's professional relationships. Knowledge of ethics gives a sound basis for dealing with difficulties that may arise in these relationships. These difficulties are often the result of conflicting values. Veterinary surgeons will have their own values, as will veterinary nurses and clients.

This is important and relevant to the role of veterinary nurses in practice. Although they are both employees and professional colleagues of veterinary surgeons, veterinary nurses may need to act as advocates for what they feel practices ought to be.

A reminder of the values at stake and the use of decision-making tools will help the veterinary nurse to work through these difficulties. Ethical professionalism requires the veterinary nurse to be knowledgeable, intelligent, patient and able to compromise, without devaluing what is at stake.[27] Professional ethics can assist the veterinary nurse to defend the professional values that ought to be defended, and change those that need to be changed.

Ethical reasoning is not easy, but done properly it is better than being rule bound and unquestioning. It signifies personal maturity and hallmarks professionalism.

THE NEED FOR VETERINARY NURSING ETHICS

Virtually everything that veterinary nurses do in their professional life reflects an ethical choice. In the current context, veterinary nursing ethics relates to what veterinary nurses do in practice. Veterinary nursing ethics is important and inescapable, because it is often far from obvious how veterinary nurses should act.[11] Ethics is complex and difficult because people have conflicting beliefs and values.

In spite of these difficulties, ethical knowledge is useful in professional practice. It is also necessary because without it, reasoning may be abstract, confusing, inconsistent and possibly unworkable. In their personal lives, veterinary nurses will use moral reasoning in everyday decision-making. Most people do this, as amoral individuals are seldom encountered. Most people are capable of recognising, and dealing with, moral situations as part of everyday life. Intuition and upbringing teaches individuals how to think and act, especially if they have been taught good principles, such as 'do not lie' 'do not steal' and so on. Moral reasoning is an essential component of life because we live in a society with other people.

There are situations where conscious practical decisions may be made without an intuitive basis.

Box 13.14

For example, some people choose to be vegetarians because they feel animals should not be used as a source of food, or do not use cosmetics that have been tested on animals.

These choices may be considered as ethical by those who make them, because they have based their decisions on how they value animals. For others who do not share these values, eating meat and using cosmetics tested on animals would not be unethical.

There are, however, more difficult situations, such as those encountered in veterinary nursing practice. In practice, the veterinary nurse relates to animals, whose health status means that they require professional help, and also to their owners. This relationship is a human interaction and highly individual. To base ethical reasoning purely on intuition would create difficulties, because the moral intuition that we rely on in our own everyday life is of limited use in professional practice. What is needed is a framework to assist decision-making that is grounded in an understanding of ethics.

ETHICAL FRAMEWORKS

The knowledge needed for ethical decision-making is based mainly on two classical theories, utilitarianism and deontology. These are sometimes called normative theories, as they provide a norm or standard to be applied. They are not mutually exclusive. Elements of each theory can be recognised in decision-making.

Applying these theories in practice can be made easier by focusing on the four principles that have been made famous in bioethics (commonly called health care ethics). Though the four principles have been criticised for being too superficial and limited, they are useful in reminding the veterinary nurse of the key dimensions of ethical thinking. They also provide a framework and common vocabulary for professionals who may have different ethical philosophies. Theories and principles alone will not help decision-making. It is important to gain as much information as possible, establish the facts and clarify key concepts to make sure that all those involved are talking about and addressing the same issues.[28]

Respect for autonomy, beneficence, non-maleficence and fairness are the basic tools in the application of ethics to practice. Table 13.2 illustrates the links between these ethical principles and the two ethical theories when applied in practice.

In addition, both utilitarianism and deontology make a special point of identifying how human beings should related to animals. When talking about animals, Bentham, a utilitarian, famously stated:[29]

The question is not, can they reason? Nor, can they talk? But can they suffer?

Bentham's argument is based on an animal's capacity to suffer:

... that the capacity to suffer gives a being (animal) the right to be given equal consideration.

This is supported by a contemporary philosopher who states 'that the capacity for suffering and enjoying things is a prerequisite for having interests, which must be satisfied before we speak of interests in any meaningful way'.[30]

Table 13.2

Ethical principle	Utilitarianism	Deontology
Autonomy: animals and individuals have freedoms and can make choices	On balance good outcomes are achieved by respecting animals and individuals	It is our duty to respect animals as this improves our humanity towards others
Beneficence: goodness and welfare should be promoted	The overall benefits for animals and individuals are increased	Our duty is to promote animal welfare because it will benefit the owner
Non-maleficence: animals and individuals should not be harmed unnecessarily, either physically or psychologically	This balances with promoting benefits for animals and individuals	Our duty is to avoid deliberate harm to others where possible
Justice/fairness: animals and individuals should be treated equally	The overall outcome is to achieve good for as many animals and individuals as possible	Our duty is to treat all animals equally as this is necessary in our relationship with individuals

When it came to animals, Kant, a deontologist, believed that animals should be regarded as instruments to be used by humans.[30] Animals, he argued, are not self-conscious and are there merely as a means to an end, that end is man. He did believe that man has duties to animals; these he considered to be indirect duties.

He argued that our relationship towards animals develops our humanity. For example, if a person is inhuman towards an animal, this will damage the person's humanity, which it is his duty to show towards another person. This citation from an old translation makes the point, 'for he who is cruel to animals becomes hard also in his dealings with men'. This translation goes on to say; 'We can judge the heart of a man by his treatment of animals'.[30]

PROFESSIONAL ETHICAL DECISION-MAKING

Veterinary nurses can be involved in a multitude of ethical situations. The diversity of veterinary practice and the veterinary nurse's relationship with the patient and client can contribute to a complex scenario. Professional veterinary nursing practice is based on the application of knowledge to practice. The challenge is how to make ethical knowledge meaningful, because ethical decisions should be an integral component of all practice.[31]

As individuals, we constantly make moral judgements about what we consider to be right or wrong and the best course of action to take. We seldom analyse these thoughts or actions, but use our gut instinct or intuition to decide what to do. We may justify it to ourselves by declaring that it 'just felt right' or it was 'the right thing to do'. This is acceptable and an important way of making decisions in our personal, but not professional, lives.[32] If this method is used in professional ethical decision-making, it is of limited use and could lead to unethical decisions being made.

> **Box 13.15**
>
> For example: you may be fond of mice and keep them as pets. The practice you work in has an infestation of rodents. Do you treat them as pets, or eradicate them?

The ability to make ethical decisions is essential to professional nursing practice.[33] Human nurse education includes ethics and decision-making within the curriculum. Nurses are encouraged to develop critical thinking skills and to link knowledge to practice. Students are taught to examine their personal values and beliefs, and to compare them with the values underpinning nursing care and practice. They analyse the standards of ethical behaviour in the code of professional conduct.

This integration becomes part of the nurse's framework for ethical decision-making and its implementation in nursing practice.[34]

Ethical behaviour is not only reserved for times of crisis. It is an everyday expression of commitment to the way in which human beings relate to one another and to animals. However, this is not always easy or clear cut. When presented with an ethical situation, it can either be a problem or a dilemma. A problem can be solved. Dilemmas, on the other hand, are much more difficult to resolve because they require a choice to be made between 'what seem to be two equally desirable or undesirable alternatives'.[35] The outcome of the chosen option can leave the nurse feeling dissatisfied and uncomfortable. The following example illustrates this point.

Box 13.16

An emaciated and flea-infested dog has been brought into the practice you work in. The client claims that the dog belongs to a friend who is too unwell to accompany the dog. The client requests euthanasia for the patient stating that the owner is unable to look after the dog. The veterinarian agrees to the request but you are very unhappy with this decision. The dog is euthanased.

You feel that by spending more time in finding out about the owner of the dog, and the circumstances surrounding this case, the dog could be treated and maybe re-homed. The other possibility is that the owner will miss the dog.

This scenario suggests that if the nurse had more time to consider the situation, and gather more information, the outcome could be different. The dog would be alive, either in a new home or back with its owner.

Professional accountability requires nurses to be clear in their directions, they need to know what is expected of them. This involves the ability to make decisions.[21]

ETHICAL DECISION-MAKING TOOLS

Veterinary nurses make decisions based on several issues, reflecting areas of knowledge that are taken into consideration. These may include knowledge of the animal's anatomy and physiology, the psychology of animal behaviour, the effect of drug actions and previous experience of treating similar cases. These represent different standpoints. One particular standpoint, for example the animal's health or the circumstances of the owner, may form the basis of the decision.

Models of ethical decision-making represent the various approaches that might be taken. These models are useful in helping to establish the important issues of each case. They examine the values and interests of the animals and people involved. Nurses will use their own knowledge of ethics, practical experiences, moral sensitivity and personal motivation to arrive at an ethical decision and act on it.[34]

The nursing process is a problem-solving tool used by nurses in everyday practice. The steps are established and clear, and could be used as a tool to work through an ethical situation.

Assessment

The first stage in assessment is to clarify the issues and establish the facts. It is necessary to consider what is at stake, for example, who should be the focus of attention, the animal, the owner or both? Ask questions to help sort out fact from assumption and important from irrelevant information. Not all situations encountered in veterinary practice will be predominantly ethical. Some will be clinical. When the situation is of an ethical nature it could be mainly legal and to a lesser extent ethical or vice versa. This could lead to difficulty in the decision-making process because of the potential conflict that can arise between the legal and ethical issues. Professionally, the nurse must work within the law.

Planning

Once the assessment has established the facts, a plan of action can be formulated. The outcome of the action, both immediately and long-term, must be clear. Should the goal of the plan be directed at a good outcome for the majority, this would be a utilitarian approach, while a goal focused on what is the ethical duty of the key player would be a

Table 13.3

Steps of the nursing process decision-making tool	Areas of knowledge to be considered	Questions to be considered
Assessment	Clarify the issues. Establish the facts consider: ethical theories legal issues code of conduct clinical knowledge local policies	What is the key issue, the animal, owner or both? What ethical values are at stake? What ethical principles need to be considered? Is the treatment proposed based on evidence?
Planning	Experience of staff members. Consider: past experience diversity of experience consider alternatives immediate and long term goal decision-making	Who in the team can make the decision? Veterinary nurse alone? Veterinary surgeon alone? Or is it a team effort?
Implementation	Communication Consider: the values the concepts ethical principles lines of communication clear, unambiguous course of action	Is the basis of the decision clear to all? Is the decision acceptable to all? If not, why not?
Evaluation	Gather the facts following the implementation question those involved reflect	Who acted? Was it acceptable to all? How do they feel? Should the same decision be made again?

deontological approach. To help with the plan, members of staff may have experiences from similar situations that can be sought. Planning is a skilful undertaking, requiring knowledge, practical experience and skills. Communication and clinical skills are necessary, because once the plan has been made it should be clear and unambiguous. However, having a good plan and experience cannot prevent or protect against the unexpected. Professionals need to be flexible, resourceful and able to alter a plan.

Implementation

Implementing the plan can be the most difficult step in the process. It requires confidence and courage to act upon what has been decided. It is not without risk. What if something had not been considered in the planning stage, or more information became known while implementing the plan? Ethical deliberation and judgement will be necessary in the management of changes in implementation.

Evaluation

Evaluation is an assessment of the consequences of the action. It involves finding out if the actual consequences were different from the intended outcome. It must establish if the outcome is ethically acceptable and stands up to scrutiny. It requires staff to reflect on their actions and feelings at the time, and after the event. This feedback is a learning opportunity. If the action did achieve a good outcome, it can be used again and may be considered as an example of good practice. If, however, the outcome is not good, the process of working out why this happened is a learning tool.

Consistent ethical decision-making in the workplace will earn respect for the veterinary nurse as a knowledgeable, thinking professional who can resolve ethical situations related to specific areas of practice.[34]

ADVOCACY

Ethical professional practice will from time to time require veterinary nurses to act on behalf of the animals, and possibly the owners, in their care. Their roles as advocates for animals may lie between the animals' best interests and the wishes of the owner. The role may require representation for the animal against the veterinary surgeon.

Advocacy is a difficult role to adopt, and it is fraught with problems. However, human nursing has debated the concept, and it may be helpful to consider some of the difficulties highlighted by this debate.

There is a wealth of literature on this subject, written by nurses, nurse philosophers and non-nurses writing about nursing. Many writers cite the ambiguity of the concept, and many suggest that it should be treated with caution, debated and examined, before it is accepted and implemented into the nurse's role. As a concept within human nursing, advocacy has been around since the 1970s (mainly in North America). The International Council of Nursing (ICN) included advocacy in its 1973 code, and at the same time dropped from this code the requirement that nurses should be obedient to doctors. The United Kingdom Central Council for Nurses, Midwives and Health Visitors (UKCC) introduced the concept in a document explaining accountability in 1989. This document clearly states 'that the practitioner will accept a role as advocate on behalf of his or her patient/client'.[36]

The term advocacy is used and defined in various ways. Descriptions range from counsellor, therapist and representative to rights advocate.[37] It is important to distinguish between an independent and a professional advocate.[38] There are different types of people who may undertake advocacy. For example, a legally trained person will represent a person's legal rights, or an organisation may advocate for a group with common status (e.g. Age Concern).

Initially, the UKCC did not give any guidance as to how nurses should act as patients' advocates; however, in a document produced in 1996 the following advice was given:[39]

Advocacy can be achieved by:

- providing information,
- making patients feel confident that they can make their own decisions, and
- providing support if patients refuse treatment or care or withdraw their consent.

Advocacy is concerned with promoting and protecting the interests of patients or clients.

Advocacy within human nursing has taken root, but there is still controversy. Many nurses welcome it, while some outside the profession are critical of how nurses can be advocates.[40] The benchmark for human nurses is the advice from the NMC, which implies that advocacy is part of the professional nurse's role.

The RCVS Guide to Professional Conduct for Veterinary Nurses does not explicitly state that veterinary nurses are required to be advocates. However, it could be argued that it is implied within the following statements.[41]

- They shall act at all times in the best interests of the animals, while taking into consideration the wishes of the owner/keeper and employer, and in such a manner as to justify the trust and confidence of the public and to uphold the good standing of the veterinary profession.
- Veterinary nurses should be mindful of their responsibility to report to their employer any circumstances where the health and safety of staff or animals is put at risk.

Like human nursing, advocacy and the role of the veterinary nurse can be controversial. Who does the veterinary nurse act as advocate for, the animal, the owner or both? It would seem from the above statements that veterinary nurses must advocate

Box 13.17

For example, the owner of a flea-infested dog refuses to have flea treatment, arguing that fleas are living creatures and should not be killed. You advocate that the dog's health will be undermined if the infestation is not treated, giving sound evidence, treatment options and at the same time promoting the welfare of the dog.

for both, but this begs the question, against whom must they advocate? In human nursing, it has been argued that nurses advocate against the dominant professional group, that is, medical staff. This implies that this group of professionals is not representing the interests of their patients or clients. This is a false assumption. Health care is multidisciplinary and patients/clients benefit when all health professionals work together to promote their interests. Research found that when human nurses were acting as patients' advocates, there was no power struggle with other professionals.[42] In fact, the opposite was true. Nurses were quite clear in their thinking that the environment in which the care is situated, and in which advocacy occurs, should be one which values all the contributions made, and which puts patients, rather than any member of the health team, at the powerful centre of care.

Within veterinary nursing practice there is still the opportunity for controversy and ethical dilemma. When there is a conflict between the interests of the animal and the wishes of the owner, what should be the veterinary nurse's role? The primary focus of veterinary nursing care is the patient, whose interests and well-being should be paramount. The client should be treated in an ethical and professional way, as outlined in the veterinary nurses' guide. Working together to come to a favourable compromise, which respects the animal's interests and the owner's wishes, should be the aim of decision-making. Advocacy is not about winning, it is about professionally representing the interests of those involved.

Advocacy can be risky, as the outcome can be difficult to predict. Research in human nursing found that nurses who were acting as advocates had sound professional identity, high levels of self-esteem and self–confidence, and were prepared to accept the risks associated with advocacy. A key factor for the nurses in the research group was having a clear focus of nursing accountability. They were also personally and professionally secure.[42]

CONCLUSION

The way forward for veterinary nursing is to focus on developing a professional identity. This will give practitioners a sense of professional confidence and worth. However, this has to be earned and developed, through education and practice, always focusing on the fact that professionalism is linked with ethical practice. Ethical practice is not a one-off exercise; it is continuous and must be displayed in all professional situations. This includes relationships with patients, clients and professional colleagues. Professionalism requires the veterinary nurse to be accountable for actions and omissions. It also requires the veterinary nurse to accept that being a professional may seem risky and onerous. This can be challenging. It is worth remembering that knowledge will give the veterinary nurse power to question the employer, usually a veterinary surgeon or other veterinary nurse.

This chapter has offered an introduction to frameworks and useful tools to guide and assist the veterinary nurse in being ethically professional in practice. Veterinary nurses can learn from some of the developments made in human nursing. After all, human nurses have learned, and will no doubt continue to learn, from other professional disciplines within and outside health care.

References

1. Burnard P, Chapman C. Professional and ethical issues in nursing. 3rd edn. London: Bailliere Tindall; 2003:2.

2. Carr-Saunders AM, Wilson PA. The professions. London: Frank Cass; 1964.

3. Hall C. Who controls the nursing profession? The role of the professional association. Occasional paper. Nursing Times 1973; 69(23):89–92.

4. Nursing and Midwifery Council. An NMC guide for students of nursing and midwifery. London: UKCC; 2002.

5. Nursing and Midwifery Council Code of professional conduct 2004. Online. Available: http://www.nmc-uk.org/nmc/main/publications/Codeofprofconductfinal.pdf. 9 Jun 2005.

6. Reeves M, Orford J. Fundamental aspects of legal, ethical and professional issues in nursing. Salisbury: Quay books; 2002.

7. Keogh J. Professionalisation of nursing: development, difficulties and solutions. Journal of Advanced Nursing 1997; 25:302–308.

8. Quinn CA, Smith MD. The professional commitment: issues and ethics in nursing. London: WB Saunders Co; 1987.

9. Joel LA. Kelly's dimensions of professional nursing. 9th edn. New York: McGraw-Hill; 1999.

10. Kelly LY. Dimensions of professional nursing. 9th edn. New York: McGraw-Hill; 1999: 193.

11. Tannenbaum J. Veterinary ethics. Animal welfare, client relations, competition and collegiality. 2nd edn. St Louis: Mosby; 1995.

12. Tschudin V, Ethics in nursing: the caring relationship. 2nd edn. London: Heinemann; 1990.

13. Curtain L, Flathery MJ. Nursing ethics, theories and pragmatics. New York: Prentice-Hall; 1982.

14. Coletta SS. Values clarification in nursing: why? American Journal of Nursing. December 1978; 2057.

15. Uustal DB. Values clarification in nursing: application to practice. American Journal of Nursing. December 1978; 2058–2063.

16. Rath LE, Harmin M, Simon S. Values and teaching. Colombus: Merrill Books; 1966.

17. Beauchamp TL, Childress JK. Principles of biomedical ethics. 3rd edn. New York: OUP; 1989.

18. Gillon R. Principles of health care ethics. Chichester: Wiley; 1994.

19. Thiroux J. Ethics: theory and practice. London: Collier McMillan; 1986.

20. Mc Gann S. The development of nursing as an accountable profession. In: Watson R, ed. Accountability in nursing practice. London: Chapman-Hall; 1995:18–29.

21. Walsh M. Nursing frontiers: accountability and boundaries of care. Oxford: Butterworth: 2000.

22. Pearson A, Vaughan B. Nursing models for practice. Oxford: Butterworth; 1986.

23. Bergman R. Accountability–definition and dimension. International Nursing Review 1981; 28(2):53–59.

24. Hancock HC. Professional responsibility: implications for nursing practice within the realms of cardio-thoracics. Journal of Advanced Nursing 1997; 24:1054–1060.

25. Bristol Royal Infirmary Inquiry. Final report. Online. Available http://www.bristol-inquiry.org.uk 9 Jun 2005.

26. Rutgers LJE. The use of the reflective equilibrium method in teaching animal ethics and veterinary ethics. Online. Available: http://www.ensaia.u-nancy.fr/bioethics/workshop/pdf/Rutgers.pdf 9 Jun 2005.

27. Seedhouse D. Ethics, the heart of health care. 2nd edn. Chichester: Wiley; 1998.

28. Cribb A. The ethical dimension. In: Tingle J, CribbA, eds. Nursing law and ethics. Oxford: Blackwell Science; 1995.

29. Singer P. A utilitarian view. In: Kushe H, Singer P, eds. Bioethics, an anthology. Oxford: Blackwell; 1999:56.

30. Kushe H, Singer P, eds. Bioethics, an anthology. Oxford: Blackwell; 1999:459–470.

31. Greipp ME. Greipp's model of ethical decision making. Journal of Advanced Nursing 1992;17:734–738.

32. Thompson IE, Melia KM, Boyd KM. Nursing ethics. 4th edn. Edinburgh: Churchill Livingstone; 2000.

33. Fry ST, Johnstone MJ. Ethics in nursing practice. A guide to ethical decision making. 2nd edn. Oxford: Blackwell Science; 2002.

34. Fry ST, Johnstone MJ. Ethics in nursing practice. A guide to ethical decision making. 2nd edn. Oxford: Blackwell Science; 2002:55–62.

35. Johnstone MJ. Bioethics: a nursing perspective. 3rd edn. Sydney: Harcourt Saunders; 1999:177.

36. United Kingdom Central Council. Exercising accountability. London: UKCC; 1989:12.

37. Chadwick R, Tadd W. Ethics and nursing practice: a case study approach. Basingstoke: Macmillan;1992.

38. Gates B. Advocacy: A nurse's guide. London: Scutari; 1994.

39. UKCC Guidelines for professional practice. London: UKCC; 1996.

40. Allmark P. Do nurses have a special claim to be patient advocates? In: Tadd W, ed Ethical and professional issues in nursing perspectives from Europe. Basingstoke: Palgrave; 2004.

41. Royal College of Veterinary Surgeons.List of Veterinary Nurses. London: RCVS; 2005.

42. Snowball J. Asking nurses about advocating for patients: 'reactive' and 'proactive' accounts. Journal of Advanced Nursing 1996; 24: 67–75.

Glossary of terms

Adverse drug reaction A reaction that is harmful and unintended and which occurs at doses normally used in animals for the prophylaxis, diagnosis or treatment of disease or the modification of physiological function.

Adverse effects Adverse effects refers to the avoidable pain, suffering and distress caused by a procedure.

Alternatives This refers to use of research methods that use non-sentient material, instead of conscious living vertebrates, and include: plants, micro-organisms, developmental stages of vertebrates, in-vitro methods, human studies computer and mathematical models.

Animal-based research Any scientific investigation involving the use of animals or tissues derived from animals.

Animal Procedures Committee A national advisory body offering advice to the Home Secretary on policy and practice issues relating to Animals (Scientific Procedures) Act 1986 and responsible for investigating and advising upon issues that it feels are of concern to the public.

Animal rights The concept that states all conscious animals have an inherent value or built in worth arising from an individual's conscious experience of its own life and the importance of that experience to the animal itself.

Animals (Scientific Procedures) Act 1986 The legislation that governs the use of animals in scientific research in the UK, but generally not those used in clinical based studies.

Certificate of designation The licensing that regulates the place in which regulated animal-based can be carried out and where research animals can be bred and housed.

Certificate holder The person who holds the certificate of designation and ultimately carries the responsibility for what occurs in the establishment.

Clinical trials The testing of products or devices 'in practice' or 'in the real world' that have been developed through regulated research. Clinical trials are often conducted as part of routine clinical veterinary practice.

Codes of practice Under the Animals (Scientific Procedures) Act 1986 there are a number of codes of practice that provide recommendations on appropriate standards of housing and care for laboratory animals. For example, the codes of practice for the 'Housing and care of animals used in scientific procedures' and 'Housing and care for animals in designated breeding and supply establishments'.

Currency A system in which the things that it comprises share the same qualities and quantities and so are directly comparable with each other.

Equal consideration of interests An ethical principle that states that in deciding whether a particular use of an animal is right or wrong, we should give equal weight to the interests of the animals involved as we would to our own interests if we were used in the same way.

Genetically modified animals Animals that have had their genetic makeup deliberately altered by having genetic material either removed or added from another organism resulting in a permanent change in one or more of its characteristics.

Harmful mutations A genetic mutation that can or does potentially compromise the health or well-being of the animal affected.

Humane Inflicting the minimum of pain and distress.

Humane endpoints This refers to the predetermined point at which the level of adverse effects exceeds what is considered to be justifiable and results in the animals being immediately euthanised.

Informed consent The confirmation of an owner's willingness to participate in a particular trial. This confirmation should only be sought after information has been given about the owner's rights and responsibilities, about the risk and inconveniences related to the investigation and the objectives and benefits thereof.

Lay person A person without professional or specialised knowledge.

Local ethical review committee A local advisory body within each establishment that provides independent ethical advice on project applications and the standards of animal care and welfare.

Named animal care and welfare officer The individual(s) responsible for the day-to-day care of the animals within a research establishment.

Named veterinary surgeon The veterinary surgeon that is responsible for providing advice on the health and welfare of the animals within the research establishment.

Non-regulated research Animal-based research that is NOT regulated by legislation, e.g. 1986 Animals (Scientific Procedures) Act, as it is NOT considered to cause unavoidable pain, suffering and distress to any of the animals involved. However, non-regulated research is often regulated at a local (individual institution) level by their own welfare and research committees.

Placebo Substance given/procedure performed that has no intrinsic therapeutic value.

Production animals Animals that are farmed in some way for their products, e.g. beef and dairy cattle, sheep, pigs, chickens, fish and rabbits, etc.

Project licence The licence required for conducting a programme of research, which explicitly states the specific procedures and species that can be used and the place where the whole programme of work is to be carried out.

Protected animal This refers to those non-human living vertebrates and *Octopus vulgaris* used in regulated research in the UK.

Quality of life The concept that an individual has a right to live free from harm, abuse, and exploitation, and so experience all aspects of life such as pain, pleasure, fear, joy and suffering.

Regulated procedure Any procedure carried out on a protected animal under the 1986 Animals (Scientific Procedures) Act.

Regulated research Animal-based research that is controlled and governed by legislation, e.g. 1986 Animals (Scientific Procedures) Act, as it is deemed to cause unavoidable pain, suffering and distress to the animals involved. Regulated research makes up the majority of animal-based research in the UK.

Schedule 1 The part of the 1986 Animals (Scientific Procedures) Act responsible for regulating how laboratory animals are euthanised.

Schedule 2 The part of the 1986 Animals (Scientific Procedures) Act responsible for regulating where laboratory animals are sourced from.

Scientific establishment The site of the majority of regulated animal-based research that conducts studies for either or both human and animal benefit. For example, pharmaceutical companies, contract research laboratories, agro-chemical companies, universities and government research facilities.

Severity banding The banding used to classify the severity of each specific procedure within a project and the overall severity of the project itself.

Speciesism The act of assigning different values or rights to beings on the basis of their biological species, rather than according to the characteristics they possess, such as the ability to suffer.

Utilitarianism The ethical principle of doing 'the greatest good for the greatest number while causing the least harm' and involves weighing up the costs and benefits of a particular course of action or situation.

Please read the following scenarios and reach a decision about what you would do/think in a similar situation. There are no answers to this, as they are a test of your personal ethical principles.

The ethical dilemma

An owner brings in a heavily pregnant cat and informs the vet that she cannot cope with a litter of kittens. The vet estimates the pregnancy to be at the seven week stage. The owner wishes to have the cat spayed otherwise she will have to take her to a cat rescue shelter. The vet agrees to carry out the operation. The theatre nurse does not wish to be involved as she has strong views on terminating pregnancies. Should she be forced to assist?

A cruelty case?

A dog is brought in as an emergency bleeding from a neck wound. It has obviously been caused by a severe rope burn. The dog survives major surgery to repair deep lacerations. The vet asks you to contact the RSPCA to investigate the case. They agree to do this but decide not to prosecute the owner as he had actually brought the dog to the veterinary surgeon. The case would therefore be unlikely to end in prosecution. Two things to think about – were you within your rights to report the owner to the RSPCA? And do you think that the owner should have been prosecuted?

RTA – should you help?

A nurse is driving home when the car in front hits a Shar-Pei dog. He leaps out and offers to assess the situation. The dog is haemorrhaging from its mouth and seems to have fractured its right fore radius. The nurse tries to apply a splint to the limb then offers to transport the animal to the practice where he works having phoned the vet on call. Unfortunately the dog dies on the way to the surgery. The owner complains and seeks compensation from the practice saying that the few minutes it took to apply the splint made the difference between life and death. What would you do in a similar situation?

Negligence?

The nurse in charge of in-patients is asked by the vet to give insulin at 12.00 to a cat. The nurse injects the cat on time, however forgets to write it on the card and goes off for lunch. The vet checks the card at 12.15 and thinks that the insulin has not been given and repeats the dose. The cat collapses and goes into a hypoglycaemic coma. Luckily it is spotted and treated, but the cat is left with brain damage. Whose fault is it?

Professional misconduct and whistle-blowing

A nurse on duty on Christmas day receives a phone call from a client whose dog is having problems whelping. After taking down the details she telephones the vet on duty who asks her to tell the clients to bring the dog to the surgery. The vet and the clients arrive at the same time and after examining the dog the vet decides it requires a caesarean. He informs the clients to call back in an hour and asks the nurse to prepare for surgery. It is at this point that the nurse notices that the vet is slurring his words, appears unsteady on his feet and smells strongly of alcohol. What are your options?

Duty to follow veterinary surgeon's instructions

A locum vet has arrived at the practice and is doing all the routine ops. You have prepared carprofen for all the bitch spays, as this is normal practice procedure. You ask the vet if he would like you to give the injections and he says 'no, don't bother they don't need that'. You decide to give it anyway. The vet discovers this when he looks at the prepared bill for one of the bitch spays. He is not very pleased. Should you have done this?

Insurance fraud?

A cat has been hospitalised for the past three days for investigation of polydipsia and weight loss. A routine biochemistry profile has been performed but the main clinical finding is an enlarged thyroid. You have been asked to discharge the cat and to book it in for a thyroidectomy in 10 days time. When you print off the bill you notice that the client has been charged for a T4 estimation. You know that this was not done. When you ask the vet in charge of the case he says 'Don't worry about that, the cat is insured'. Should you contact the insurance company?

Does it matter who performs surgery?

A client has brought a cat in for removal of a mammary tumour. He is a regular client who usually sees one of the senior partners. A nurse goes through the consent form with him and explains all the risks involved with the procedure. Unfortunately the cat dies under anaesthetic. The client subsequently discovers that one of the assistant vets performed the surgery. He complains because he was under the impression that his regular vet would be operating and had not been told otherwise. Does he have a legitimate grievance?

Explaining risk to clients

A client brings in a six month old cross breed for spaying before her first season. The client had pre-

viously seen a nurse who had discussed the advantages of spaying a bitch prior to the first season. The same nurse carefully goes through the consent form with the client and explains fully the anaesthetic risk before asking him to sign. Surgery is uneventful; the client and dog go home happy. Eight months later the client is facing a huge bill for referral to a urogenital specialist as the bitch has become incontinent. Was this truly informed consent?

Performing procedures not on the consent form

A Cavalier King Charles Spaniel was presented with a grass seed in its left front foot. The grass seed was removed under sedation and the area around the site of entry was clipped and cleaned. The nurse noticed that the nails were rather long and decided to trim them. Unfortunately she cut one of the nails too short but managed to stop the bleeding. Five days later the client returned with the dog that now had an infection in that nail. The owner refused to pay the bill, as she had not asked for the nails to be cut. Does she have a point?

Who can take a blood sample from a horse?

A qualified small animal nurse goes to work at an equine referral hospital. She has had her own horses and has worked as a groom. On her second day the vet demonstrates how to take a blood sample from a horse and subsequently asks her to take blood samples on her own. Is she breaking the law?

Qualitative research

A nurse wants to perform a piece of qualitative research to find out if clients within the practice are satisfied with the way their pets are euthanased. She plans to interview them within two days of the event. What are the ethical considerations for this piece of research?

Quantitative research

A nurse wants to perform a piece of quantitative research to look at the effect of analgesia on recovery of rabbits post operatively. She plans to perform a randomised control trial where every alternate rabbit is given post-operative analgesia. What are the ethical considerations for this piece of research?

Blood donors

A stray cat is brought into the practice and instead of finding it a home the practice decides to keep it as a blood donor. As a veterinary nurse you are worried that the practice may be breaking the law by doing this.

Buying horses

A client buys a horse from a dealer. The vet examines it and it is sound, however, the horse develops behaviour problems within a few days. A nurse has studied equine behaviour and offers to give advice. By the time that the client decides that her advice is not working it is too late to return the horse.

Veterinary nurses and the Veterinary Surgeons Act 1966

Introduction

1. Under the Veterinary Surgeons Act 1966 the general rule is that only a veterinary surgeon may practise veterinary surgery. There are, however, a number of exceptions to this rule, and two of them concern veterinary nurses. This note explains the law as it applies to them.

Definition of veterinary surgery

2. Veterinary surgery as defined in the Act 'means the art and science of veterinary surgery and medicine and, without prejudice to the generality of the foregoing, shall be taken to include:

   a) the diagnosis of diseases in, and injuries to, animals including tests performed on animals for diagnostic purposes;

   b) the giving of advice based upon such diagnosis;

   c) the medical or surgical treatment of animals; and

   d) the performance of surgical operations on animals'.

What can be done by people other than veterinary surgeons

3. Schedule 3 to the Act allows anyone to give first aid in an emergency for the purpose of saving life and relieving suffering. The owner of an animal, or a member of the owner's household or employee of the owner, may also give it minor medical treatment. There are a number of other exceptions to the general rule, mainly relating to farm animals, in addition to the exceptions which apply to veterinary nurses. These are explained below.

What can be done by veterinary nurses

4. Veterinary nurses, like anyone else, may give first aid and look after animals in ways which do not involve acts of veterinary surgery. In addition, veterinary nurses may do things specified in Paragraphs 6 and 7 of Schedule 3 to the Veterinary Surgeons Act 1966 as amended by the Veterinary Surgeons Act 1966 (Schedule 3 Amendment) Order 2002. The text of these paragraphs is set out in the annex below.

Listed veterinary nurses

5. Paragraph 6 applies to veterinary nurses whose names are entered on the list maintained by RCVS. They may administer 'any medical treatment or any minor surgery (not involving entry into a body cavity)' under veterinary direction.

6. The animal must be under the care of a veterinary surgeon and the treatment must be carried out at his or her direction. The veterinary surgeon must be the employer of the veterinary nurse or be acting on behalf of the nurse's employer.

7. The directing veterinary surgeon must be satisfied that the veterinary nurse is qualified to carry out the treatment or surgery. RCVS will advise from time to time on veterinary nursing qualifications which veterinary surgeons should recognise.

8. All Listed veterinary nurses (VNs) are qualified to administer medical treatment or minor surgery (not involving entry into a body cavity), under veterinary direction, to all the species which are commonly kept as companion animals, including exotic species so kept. Unless they hold further qualifications they

are not qualified to treat the equine species, wild animals or farm animals. Listed veterinary nurses who hold the RCVS Certificate in Equine Veterinary Nursing (EVNs) are qualified to administer medical treatment or minor surgery (not involving entry into a body cavity), under veterinary direction, to any of the equine species – horses, asses and zebras.

9. A veterinary nurse should only carry out a particular act of veterinary surgery if she or he is competent to do so and has the necessary experience to deal with any problems which may arise. Where appropriate, a veterinary surgeon should be available to respond to a request for help. A veterinary nurse may only carry out acts of veterinary surgery under the direction of a veterinary surgeon, who is accountable for what is done and should ensure that he/she is covered by professional indemnity insurance.

Student veterinary nurses

10. Paragraph 7 applies to student veterinary nurses. A student veterinary nurse is someone enrolled for the purpose of training as a veterinary nurse at an approved training and assessment centre (VNAC) or veterinary practice approved by such a centre (TP). This does not include those who are undertaking the BVNA Pre-Veterinary Nursing Access Course.

11. A student veterinary nurse may administer 'any medical treatment or any minor surgery (not involving entry into a body cavity)' under veterinary nurses' veterinary direction.

12. The animal must be under the care of a veterinary surgeon and the treatment must be carried out at his/her direction. The veterinary surgeon must be the employer of the veterinary nurse or be acting on behalf of the nurse's employer.

13. The treatment or minor surgery must be carried out in the course of the student veterinary nurse's training. In the view of RVCS, such work should be undertaken only for the purpose of learning and consolidating new skills.

14. The treatment or surgery must be supervised by a veterinary surgeon or a Listed veterinary

nurse. In the case of surgery the supervision must be direct, continuous and personal.

15. In the view of the RCVS, a veterinary surgeon or Listed veterinary nurse can only be said to be supervising if they are present on the premises and able to respond to a request for assistance if needed. 'Direct, continuous and personal' supervision requires the supervisor to be present and giving the student nurse his/her undivided personal attention.

Medical treatment and minor surgery

16. The Act does not define 'any medical treatment or any minor surgery (not involving entry into a body cavity)'. Ultimately it would be for the courts to decide what these words mean.

17. The procedures which veterinary nurses are specifically trained to carry out include the following:
- administer medication by mouth, topically, by the rectum, by inhalation or by subcutaneous, intramuscular or intravenous injection;
- administer other treatments, including oral, intravenous and subcutaneous rehydration, other fluid therapy, catheterisation, cleaning and dressing of surgical wounds, treatment of abscesses and ulcers, application of external casts, holding and handling viscera when assisting in operations and cutaneous suturing;
- prepare animals for anaesthesia and assist in the administration and termination of anaesthesia, including premedication, analgesia and intubation;
- collect samples of blood, urine, faeces, skin and hair; and
- take x-rays.

Guidance on anaesthesia

18. Particular care is needed over the administration of anaesthesia. A veterinary surgeon alone should:
- assess the fitness of the animal to undergo anaesthesia;
- select and plan a suitable anaesthetic regimen;
- select any premedication; and
- administer anaesthetic if the induction dose is either incremental or to effect.

19. Provided the veterinary surgeon is physically present and immediately available for consultation, a Listed veterinary nurse may:
- administer selected sedative, analgesic or other agents before and after the operation;
- administer non-incremental anaesthetic agents on the instruction of the directing veterinary surgeon;
- monitor clinical signs and maintain an anaesthetic record; and
- maintain anaesthesia by administering supplementary incremental doses of intravenous anaesthetic agents or adjusting the delivered concentration of anaesthetic agents, under the direct instruction of the supervising veterinary surgeon.

June 2002

Annex

Paragraphs 6 and 7 of Schedule 3 to the Veterinary Surgeons Act 1966, as amended by the Veterinary Surgeons Act 1966 (Schedule 3 Amendment) Order 2002, SI 2002/1479, with effect from 10 June 2002

6. Any medical treatment or any minor surgery (not involving entry into a body cavity) to any animal by a veterinary nurse if the following conditions are complied with, that is to say:
a) the animal is, for the time being, under the care of a registered veterinary surgeon or veterinary practitioner and the medical treatment or minor surgery is carried out by the veterinary nurse at his direction;
b) the registered veterinary surgeon or veterinary practitioner is the employer or is acting on behalf of the employer of the veterinary nurse; and
c) the registered veterinary surgeon or veterinary practitioner directing the medical treatment or minor surgery is satisfied that the veterinary nurse is qualified to carry out the treatment or surgery.

In this paragraph and in paragraph 7 below:

'veterinary nurse' means a nurse whose name is entered in the list of veterinary nurses maintained by the College'.

7. Any medical treatment or any minor surgery (not involving entry into a body cavity) to any animal by a student veterinary nurse if the following conditions are complied with, that is to say:
a) the animal is, for the time being, under the care of a registered veterinary surgeon or veterinary practitioner and the medical treatment or minor sugery is carried out by the student veterinary nurse at his direction and in the course of the student veterinary nurse's training;
b) the treatment or surgery is supervised by a registered veterinary surgeon, veterinary practitioner or veterinary nurse and, in the case of surgery, the supervision is direct, continuous and personal; and
c) the registered veterinary surgeon or veterinary practitioner is the employer or is acting on behalf of the employer of the student veterinary nurse.

In this paragraph:

'student veterinary nurse' means a person enrolled under the Bye-laws made by the Council for the purpose of undergoing training as a veterinary nurse at an approved training and assessment centre or a veterinary practice approved by such a centre;

'approved training and assessment centre' means a centre approved by the Council for the purpose of training and assessing student veterinary nurses.

The Veterinary Surgeons Act 1966 (Schedule 3 Amendment) Order 1988 Statutory Instrument 1988 No. 526

Schedule 3

Excemptions from restrictions on practice of veterinary surgery

Part I

Treatment and operations which may be given or carried out by unqualified persons:

1. Any minor medical treatment given to an animal by its owner, by another member of the household of which the owner is a member or by a person in the employment of the owner.
2. Any medical or minor surgical treatment (not involving entry into a body cavity) given, otherwise than for reward, to an animal used in agriculture, as defined in the Agriculture Act 1947, by the owner of the animal or by a person engaged or employed in caring for animals so used.
3. The rendering in an emergency of first aid for the purpose of saving life or relieving pain or suffering.
4. The performance by any person of or over the age of eighteen of any of the following operations, that is to say:
   a) the castration of a male animal or the caponisation of an animal, whether by chemical means or otherwise;
   b) the docking of the tail of a lamb;
   c) the docking of the tail of a dog before its eyes are open;
   d) the amputation of the dew claws of a dog before its eyes are open.
5. The performance, by any person of the age of seventeen undergoing instruction in animal husbandry, of any operation mentioned in paragraph 4(a) or (b) above and the disbudding of a calf by any such person or by a person of over the age of eighteen undergoing such instruction, if, in each case, either of the following conditions is complied with, that is to say:
   a) the instruction in animal husbandry is given by a person registered in the register of veterinary surgeons or the supplementary veterinary register and the operation is performed under his direct, personal supervision;
   b) the instruction in animal husbandry is given at a recognised institution and the operation is performed under the direct, personal supervision of a person appointed to give such instruction at the institution.

In this paragraph 'recognised institution' means:

i) as respects Great Britain, an institution maintained or assisted (in England and Wales) by a local education authority or (in Scotland)
by an education authority or in either case an institution for the giving of further education as respects which a grant is paid by the Secretary of State or an institution recognised for the purposes of this paragraph by the Secretary of State; and
ii) as respects Northern Ireland, an agricultural college maintained by the Department of Agriculture for Northern Ireland.

Part II
Exclusions from provisions of Part I

Nothing in section 19(4)(b) of this Act shall authorise:

a) the castration of a male animal being:
   i) a horse, pony, ass or mule;
   ii) a bull, boar or goat which has reached the age of two months;
   iii) a ram which has reached the age of three months; or
   iv) a cat or dog;
b) the spaying of a cat or dog;
c) the removal (otherwise than in an emergency for the purpose of saving life or relieving pain or suffering) of any part of the antlers of a deer before the velvet of the antlers is frayed and the greater part of it has been shed;
d) the desnooding of a turkey which has reached the age of 21 days;
e) the removal of the combs of any poultry which have reached the age of 72 hours;
f) the cutting of the toes of a domestic fowl or turkey which has reached the age of 72 hours;
g) the performance of a vasectomy or the carrying out of electro-ejaculation of any animal or bird kept for production of food, wool, skin or fur or for use in the farming of land;
h) the removal of the supernumerary teats of a calf which has reached the age of three months; or
   i) the dehorning or disbudding of a sheep or goat, except the trimming of the insensitive tip of an ingrowing horn which, if left untreated, could cause pain or distress.

Revocation
3. The Veterinary Surgeons Act 1966 (Schedule 3 Amendment) Order 1982[4] is hereby revoked.

In witness whereof the Official Seal of the Minister of Agriculture, Fisheries and Food is hereunto affixed on 15th March 1988.

John Selwyn Gummer

Minister of State, Ministry of Agriculture, Fisheries and Food

Sanderson of Bowden

Minister of State, Scottish Office

14th March 1988

Peter Walker

Secretary of State for Wales

11th March 1988

Sealed with the Official Seal of the Department of Agriculture for Northern Ireland on 15th March 1988

W H Jack

Permanent Secretary

The Veterinary Surgeons Act 1966 (Schedule 3 Amendment) Order 2002

Statutory Instrument 2002 No. 1479

The Veterinary Surgeons Act 1966 (Schedule 3 Amendment) Order 2002

© Crown Copyright 2002

The text of this Internet version of the Statutory Instrument which is published by the Queen's Printer of Acts of Parliament has been prepared to reflect the text as it was made. A print version is also available and is published by The Stationery Office Limited as the The Veterinary Surgeons Act 1966 (Schedule 3 Amendment) Order 2002, ISBN 0 11 042335 6. The print version may be purchased by clicking here. Braille copies of this Statutory Instrument can also be purchased at the same price as the print edition by contacting TSO Customer Services on 0870 600 5522 or e-mail:customer.services@tso.co.uk. Further information about the publication of legislation on this website can be found by referring to the Frequently Asked Questions. To ensure fast access over slow connections, large documents have been segmented into 'chunks'. Where you see a 'continue' button at the bottom of the page of text, this indicates that there is another chunk of text available.

Statutory instruments

2002 No. 1479

Veterinary surgeons

The Veterinary Surgeons Act 1966 (Schedule 3 Amendment) Order 2002

Approved by both Houses of Parliament

Made 6th June 2002

Coming into force 10th June 2002

The Minister of Agriculture, Fisheries and Food, the Secretary of State for Scotland, the Secretary of State for Wales and the Minister of Agriculture and Rural Development for Northern Ireland, acting jointly, in exercise of the powers conferred by section 19(5) of the Veterinary Surgeons Act 1966[1] and now vested in them[2] and of all other powers enabling them in that behalf, after consultation in accordance with the said section 19(5) with the Council of the Royal College of Veterinary Surgeons and with persons appearing to them to represent interests appearing to be substantially affected, hereby make the following Order, of which a draft has been approved by a resolution of each House of Parliament:

Title and commencement

1. This Order may be cited as the Veterinary Surgeons Act 1966 (Schedule 3 Amendment) Order 2002 and shall come into force on 10th June 2002.

Amendment

2. Part I of Schedule 3 to the Veterinary Surgeons Act 1966 (exemptions from restrictions on practice of veterinary surgery)[3] shall be amended as follows –

(a) for paragraph 6[4] there shall be substituted the following paragraph –

6. Any medical treatment or any minor surgery (not involving entry into a body cavity) to any animal by a veterinary nurse if the following conditions are complied with, that is to say –

(a) the animal is, for the time being, under the care of a registered veterinary surgeon or veterinary practitioner and the medical treatment or minor surgery is carried out by the veterinary nurse at his direction;

(b) the registered veterinary surgeon or veterinary practitioner is the employer or is acting on behalf of the employer of the veterinary nurse; and

(c) the registered veterinary surgeon or veterinary practitioner directing the medical treatment or minor surgery is satisfied that the veterinary nurse is qualified to carry out the treatment or surgery.

In this paragraph and in paragraph 7 below –

'veterinary nurse' means a nurse whose name is entered in the list of veterinary nurses maintained by the College.

(b) after paragraph 6 there shall be added the following paragraph –

7. Any medical treatment or any minor surgery (not involving entry into a body cavity) to any animal by a student veterinary nurse if the following conditions are complied with, that is to say –

(a) the animal is, for the time being, under the care of a registered veterinary surgeon or veterinary practitioner and the medical treatment or minor surgery is carried out by the student veterinary nurse at his direction and in the course of the student veterinary nurse's training;

(b) the treatment or surgery is supervised by a registered veterinary surgeon, veterinary practitioner or veterinary nurse and, in the case of surgery, the supervision is direct, continuous and personal; and

(c) the registered veterinary surgeon or veterinary practitioner is the employer or is acting on behalf of the employer of the student veterinary nurse.

In this paragraph –

'student veterinary nurse' means a person enrolled under Bye-laws made by the Council for the purpose of undergoing training as a veterinary nurse at an approved training and assessment centre or a veterinary practice approved by such a centre;

'approved training and assessment centre' means a centre approved by the Council for the purpose of training and assessing student veterinary nurses.

Elliot Morley
Parliamentary Under-Secretary of State, Department for Environment, Food
and Rural Affairs
6th June 2002
Helen Liddell
Secretary of State, Scotland Office
29th May 2002
Paul Murphy
Secretary of State, Wales Office
29th May 2002
Brid Rodgers
Minister of Agriculture and Rural Development, Department of Agriculture
for Northern Ireland
29th May 2002

Explanatory note

(This note is not part of the Order)

This Order amends Schedule 3 to the Veterinary Surgeons Act 1966.

Part I of Schedule 3 to the Act (treatment and operations which may be given or carried out by unqualified persons) is amended so that a veterinary nurse (new paragraph 6) or a student veterinary nurse (new paragraph 7) may carry out any medical treatment or any minor surgery to any animal in specified circumstances.

A Regulatory Impact Assessment has been prepared and placed in the library of each House of Parliament. Copies may be obtained from the Department of Environment, Food and Rural Affairs (Animal Welfare, Branch D), 6th Floor, 1A Page Street, London SW1P 4PQ.

Notes:

[1] 1966 c. 36; 'the Ministers' referred to in section 19(5) are defined in section 27(1) as amended by paragraph 1 of Schedule 5 to S.I. 1978/272. back

[2] In the case of the Department of Agriculture for Northern Ireland, by virtue of section 40 and of paragraph 7(1) of Schedule 5 to the Northern Ireland Constitution Act 1973 (c. 36) and section 1(3) of and paragraph 2(1)(b) of Schedule 1 to, the Northern Ireland Act 1974 (c. 28).back

[3] Schedule 3 was substituted by S.I. 1988/526. back [4] Paragraph 6 was substituted by the Veterinary Surgeons Act 1966 (Schedule 3 Amendment) Order 1991, S.I. 1991/1412.back

ISBN 0 11 042335 6

Other UK SIs | Home | National Assembly for Wales Statutory Instruments | Scottish Statutory Instruments | Statutory Rules of Northern Ireland | Her Majesty's Stationery Office

We welcome your comments on this site© Crown copyright 2002 Prepared 14 June 2002

Appendix 3

Guide to Professional Conduct for Veterinary Nurses

Introduction

1. Under the Veterinary Surgeons Act 1966, the Royal College of Veterinary Surgeons is responsible for all ethical matters relating to veterinary practice within the United Kingdom. That responsibility encompasses the work of both veterinary surgeons and veterinary nurses.
2. This Code is issued to assist veterinary nurses in maintaining acceptable professional standards. Matters of concern should be raised first with their employer and thereafter if not satisfactorily resolved, with the BVNA.

General standards

3. Veterinary nurses should be mindful that they are only permitted to act under the supervision or direction of a veterinary surgeon.
4. They should be familiar with and work within the RCVS 'Guide to Professional Conduct'.
5. They are personally responsible for their own professional standards and negligence.
6. They shall act at all times in the best interests of the animal while taking into consideration the wishes of the owner/keeper and employer and in such a manner as to justify the trust and confidence of the public and to uphold the good standing of the veterinary profession.

Acknowledgements of limitations

7. Veterinary nurses are expected to maintain their professional knowledge and competence.

8. They are equally expected to acknowledge any limitations in knowledge or competence, and, where relevant, to make these known to their employer.
9. Similarly an employer should not ask a veterinary nurse to undertake any task above and beyond their known level of competence.

Relationship with veterinary colleagues

10. Veterinary nurses should co-operate fully with veterinary surgeons, assisting them in the provision of veterinary care.
11. They should encourage and help colleagues to develop their professional skills.

Conscientious objections

12. Veterinary nurses should discuss with any employer and/or prospective employer any conscientious objection which they may have to any treatment of any species of animal. Nevertheless it must be recognised that the welfare of the animal is always paramount and that there will be circumstances when this overrides any conscientious objection.

Confidentiality

13. Veterinary nurses must keep confidential any information relating to an animal or owner, an employer or fellow employee, acquired in the course of their work.
14. Such information must not be disclosed to anyone except where:
    a) They are required to do so in a court of law.

b) Where animal welfare or the wider public interest would be endangered by non disclosure.

Health and safety

15. Veterinary nurses should be mindful of their responsibility to report to their employer any circumstances where the health and safety of staff or animals is put at risk.

Promotion of products or services

16. Veterinary nurses employed in veterinary practice should not permit their professional qualification to be used as a means of promoting commercial animal related products or services to the public, nor should they allow commercial considerations to override their professional judgement.

Index